Counselling Skills for Nurses

To J.P.

Counselling Skills for Nurses

FOURTH EDITION

VERENA TSCHUDIN

BSc (Hons), RN, RM, Dip. Counselling
Counsellor, Writer, and Senior Lecturer, University of East London

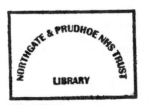
Baillière Tindall
London · Philadelphia · Toronto
Sydney · Tokyo

BAILLIÈRE TINDALL W.B. SAUNDERS
24–28 Oval Road
London NW1 7DX

The Curtis Center
Independence Square West
Philadelphia, PA 19106–3399, USA

Harcourt Brace & Company
55 Horner Avenue
Toronto, Ontario M8Z 4X6, Canada

Harcourt Brace & Company, Australia
30–52 Smidmore Street
Marrickville, NSW 2204, Australia

Harcourt Brace & Company, Japan
Ichibancho Central Building,
22–1 Ichibancho
Chiyoda-ku, Tokyo 102, Japan

First published 1982
Second edition 1987
Reprinted 1988
Third edition 1991

A catalogue record for this book is available from the British Library

ISBN 0–7020–1972–0

Typeset by Photo·graphics, Honiton, Devon
Printed in Great Britain by WBC Book Manufacturers, Bridgend, Mid Glamorgan

Contents

·········

....

Preface

When this book was first written, counselling within nursing was beginning to be taken seriously. It is now a well established discipline, at least in theory. The numbers of books on the subject testify to this, as do their frequent updates and new editions. These show not only the changing need within nursing, but also the authors' own developments and the changing understanding of the subject. This is the case also with this book.

I have tried to keep *Counselling Skills for Nurses* the basic book it has always claimed to be. This has sometimes been difficult, precisely because my understanding of the subject has changed and changes constantly. Indeed, writing a book changes one's understanding of a subject perhaps more than any other attempt to learn it. This changing is reflected in the reordering and updating of the text.

As the title suggests, this is a book for nurses. This does not mean that other health professionals are excluded, but that, in the examples used in the text, 'nurses' and 'patients' are used to describe the interactions in most instances. However, there is now much more frequent use of the term 'client' to emphasize that many counselling and helping situations are not limited to either nurses or patients: colleagues, friends and relations all need and deserve attention in a helping way.

While the theory of counselling is now acknowledged widely in nursing, the practice of it is a different matter. While this may have been due to lack of experience or skill when I first wrote the book, there is now a different reason: in the health service there is now an atmosphere in which patient contact is reduced to the absolute minimum and where human values seem to be pushed to the edges, so that counselling is tolerated but not encouraged. This is perhaps often more a perception rather than open policy. But where resources are reduced and squeezed, and time is at the highest premium, there is a question mark over the value of books such as this. Counselling led me originally into the field of ethics with the question of support for nurses who do give counselling care. It is leading me back into it, but now with the question of how to keep one's integrity and humanity in settings where these are subtly eroded and devalued.

Perhaps it is partly the publishers who keep the flame alight by printing texts such as this? My particular thanks go to Sarah James, Publisher, and the team working with her at Baillière Tindall for the support and encouragement they have provided by their warmth, genuineness and empathy.

Verena Tschudin

CHAPTER ONE

Awareness

....

'Know thyself' is one of the oldest dictums in history. But do you know yourself? Can you know yourself?

The more you are aware of yourself, the more you are aware of other people. Awareness of other people and their strengths and needs in turn helps you to be aware of these things within yourself. This is the basis of all helping, be this making a person comfortable in bed, helping someone to come to terms with illness or suffering, or enabling someone to live in more satisfying ways.

This chapter deals with different aspects of self-awareness and readers may at times feel uncomfortable if the subject matter comes rather near the bone. This does not point to a lack of awareness in readers, but is meant to enhance the readers own awareness.

Counselling and helping are possible only from a basis of self-awareness and insight into how people live and work, think and feel. This is not just theoretical knowledge, but real, raw knowledge of who you are and what you are about, and the insight gained from having listened to who and what other people are, do and say. Unless there is such a basic knowledge and awareness we cannot help others. Indeed, without awareness of ourselves we can actually damage other people. This would be a contradiction if it were not for the fact that we are all dependent on each other and affect one another by our behaviour.

There are numerous ways of developing insight and awareness of who and what we are. From psychoanalysis, astrology, intelligence tests, psychometric tests, the Myers–Briggs Type Indicator and Chinese horoscopes, to quick self-assessments in magazines and books, there is a wealth of information available on how to understand oneself better.

Any measurements that 'reveal' ourselves are only partial. They are never the truth, the whole truth and nothing but the truth. The greatness, and also the difficulty, of self-awareness

is that there is always more to a person or situation than can
be known or predicted. There is also the aspect that all life
changes constantly. Life around us changes and we change
with it, whether we want to or not. Self-awareness is therefore
a never-ending experience.

An understanding of our basic temperament can be very
helpful and may remove much pain and guilt and allow the
development of natural assertiveness. But beyond that, we are
what we allow ourselves to be. In this way we discover not only
ambiguities and discrepancies, but also meaning and purpose.

Self-awareness concerns both our inner and outer world and
the go-between world of the senses. This means knowing the
impact our body language has on others – and indeed, what
our body language actually is. It could be difficult to give a
patient bad news when you have just passed your exams and
cannot stop smiling; or to convince a relative that a loved one
is not seriously ill when you shift around on your chair and
speak in a tone that may be more appropriate in a mortuary.
Shakespeare knew, and we all know it too, that there is language in our eyes, cheeks, lips and feet, and that our 'wanton
spirits' look out from every joint and movement of our bodies.

Being aware of feelings may not be so difficult; acknowledging these feelings is much more difficult. Nurses have a
shocking capacity to learn very early to suppress feelings and
think that this is a virtue. We exhort patients and clients to
weep but do not allow ourselves to do the same. This is not
only unreasonable but dishonest and potentially harmful. By
denying part of ourselves we deny a whole (holistic) attitude
in ourselves which may transfer to patients.

Philips (1993) believes that because nurses are expected to
care for others, this makes them think of themselves as different. Their role of carer is entrenched in their personality and
that makes them very bad at caring for themselves. The professional culture seems to indicate that good nurses are able
to take anything thrown at them. We all have to adopt certain
roles which are given to us in personal and professional life.
One of the important things to learn early in any helping career
is which roles fit and which do not, which help and which
hinder, which to keep and which to discard.

A lack of self-understanding or self-acknowledgement
means that there are areas about ourselves that are unknown
to us or unaccepted by us. What we do not know about ourselves we tend not to acknowledge in others. What we deny
in ourselves we tend to deny in others. This means that we

reduce our capacity for helping. When we increase our self-understanding, we increase our capacity to help.

The senses – seeing, hearing, feeling, tasting, touching – make the link between outer and inner worlds. They convey feelings of sadness through facial expressions and make it possible for a tasty morsel to create love. Nurses are acutely aware of the importance of the senses in practice, and a conscious use of all senses can only enhance that practice.

As you allow yourself to sit and stare, and take time to be aware of yourself, you are laying the basis for being a counsellor. Counselling is not about giving the right answer, but it is about being with another person 'there where it hurts'. This means that you have a sense of that hurt because you have experienced something similar. It does not mean identifying with another, but going alongside.

Awareness is not something that we learn from books. Insights and flashes of inspiration may come from books, but awareness of oneself is learnt in daily interactions. Being aware of one's own deep feelings and being able to understand and predict one's own emotional responses leads to greater self-security. This in turn influences how we see and help our patients and clients. It is hardly surprising that patients and clients are often low in self-esteem and self-trust. When they meet these aspects in the caring staff they may be able to take the first step in recovering them for themselves.

Awareness of ourselves is strengthening, and gives us control and freedom to be that which we really are.

The person of the helper

The more we are ourselves, the more real we are as *people* generally, not only as helpers.

Those who help others are not supermen and superwomen or paragons of virtue. If they were, they would not be effective helpers. This is not to say that the lazy win. Wanting to help others demands first of all that we respect the other person for who and what she or he is and this means going beyond your own prejudices and personal limits. Helping demands an effort on our part. There is also a satisfaction in helping which is experienced at a human level but can hardly be measured. But neither do we help *in order to* get satisfaction. We help out of a deep sense of duty, of sharing with people in suffering, and perhaps out of a little acknowledged or unconscious need to be helped ourselves.

To help effectively, we have to be committed to ourselves and our own values and principles. Some of these are clear, some seem to be imposed and some are perhaps accepted without being questioned. Like nursing generally, helping is not done by rote but involves the whole of the person. This does often mean stretching boundaries and going where it hurts. Courage is not something that only soldiers need but which helpers also require. Above all, helping others means being willing to be constantly challenged by patients and clients. Our values, skills, views, models, knowledge and capacities have to be reviewed and adapted all the time. Self-awareness teaches us how to do this and when, and this in turn sharpens self-awareness and self-knowledge.

You do not become a good helper only after you have acquired all the skills. You do not have to know every model before you can help anybody. You learn by doing, and doing teaches you.

How do you see yourself as a helper? What are your reasons for wanting to learn about counselling and helping skills? You have often helped people in this way; what do *you* get out of it?

When you realize that you want to counsel, not because you are good at it but because through counselling some deep need within yourself is satisfied, then you are sincere and genuine, and that comes across to the person who is helped. This is not to say that you are an unfulfilled person, but that you have recognized and acknowledged your own needs and respond to them in the most adequate way for you yourself. When you know your true needs, and what makes you tick, then you are more free to listen to others. Or, as Rogers (1961, p. 51) said:

One way of putting this . . . is that if I can form a helping relationship to myself – if I can be sensitively aware of an acceptance toward my own feelings – then the likelihood is great that I can form a helping relationship toward another.

Self-awareness goes together with certain attitudes that are essential to helping. In a sense you have to 'be' these things to yourself before you can be them to and with others. Genuine helping happens when these elements are there. But to *be* any of these things genuinely is not easy. Helping is not just a set of skills, but a way of being, as Rogers (1980) repeatedly said.

Rogers also used 'genuineness', 'congruence' and 'realness' to describe this experience which is a coming-together of experience and awareness and communication.

Experience drove home the fact that to act consistently acceptant, for example, if in fact I was feeling annoyed or sceptical or some other non-acceptant feeling, was certain in the long run to be perceived as inconsistent or untrustworthy. I have come to recognize that being trustworthy does not demand that I be rigidly consistent but that I be dependably real. The term 'congruent' is one I have used to describe the way I would like to be. By this I mean that whatever feeling or attitude I am experiencing would be matched by my awareness of that attitude. When this is true, then I am a unified or integrated person in that moment, and hence I can be whatever I deeply am. This is a reality which I find others experience as dependable. (Rogers, 1961, p. 51)

Rogers was the first person to describe the discipline of counselling as it is practised today. In his classic book *On Becoming a Person* (1961) he describes many aspects of helping in philosophical rather than purely practical terms and reading this text has helped many students of counselling to arrive at a clearer understanding of what might be involved in this kind of work.

To be consistent in a helping relationship demands many of the skills described later. It also asks of you as helper that you use all the communication skills at your disposal. But more than that, consistency of behaviour denotes a large measure of self-awareness. When you know yourself, then you are less likely to be put off, found out, or dishonest with others. It demands awareness of yourself, but it also demands that you share that awareness in the relationship. Nurse (1980, p. 45) puts this into context:

When we are at our place of work, occupying a particular position in a social structure, it is all too easy to take refuge in our professional role as tutor, midwife, nursing officer or whatever it may be, and to use that role as a means of protecting ourselves or as a substitute for effectiveness.

It is possible to take refuge in a perceived role: that of being kind, or caring or just. These may be acceptable ways of being, and they are very good ones, but only if they are 'real' to the person concerned. When you are able to identify the discrepancies in your life, particularly those that affect your ability to help others, then you become a more genuine and more consistent person.

When I am 'in-place', there is a reasonable convergence between my professed values and how I actually live, between how I think and how I actually live, between how I see my behaviour from inside and how it looks to others from outside. My living testifies to what my values are. To the extent that there is significant division between inner and outer, I am not wholly in my actions; I am divided within myself, and in the end must be uncertain who I am and what I am about. (Mayeroff, 1971, p. 50)

Only when you are not trying to be 'somebody' but are simply yourself can you be trustworthy, dependable and consistent, and only then will you be seen as such by the client. The next sections elaborate on these points.

Accepting

You can often hear phrases like 'I can accept him making unreasonable demands on me when he is tired, but I cannot accept that he smacks the children'.

We cannot accept others piecemeal: 'This bit of you is OK but that bit is not'. We may not like what we encounter, but a person is all of a person, warts and all.

It is almost impossible to be totally acceptable; few people are that aware or that saintly. Accepting means, however, that we become ever more aware of ourselves in order to be more aware of others.

Accepting another person without judgement may occasionally seem incredible to clients. Those who have lost self-esteem see the world through the eyes of that loss. To meet someone who is totally and unconditionally accepting is so opposed to this image that it may seem incredible, even ridiculous: 'You must be really stupid to care for someone like me'. It is in such instances that the genuineness of the helper's character comes through. When a constancy of behaviour is evident, clients may eventually have to believe that it can be true, with the result that it may provide the basis for a self-acceptance which may change the world for that person.

Respecting

To be respectful is one of the fundamental characteristics of helpers. Egan (1994, p. 51) says that 'respect is such a fundamental notion that it eludes definition' and then goes on to describe aspects of respect. First of all, he says that it 'means prizing people simply because they are human'. This means being available to patients and clients, working with them rather than judging them, keeping the focus on their agenda, trusting the constructive forces that are there in them, and expecting them to do whatever is necessary to handle their problems in living more effectively. This can sometimes be painful for them, because it is easier for clients to have their problems solved for them than to solve them themselves. But real helping means being there alongside the personal pain rather than taking it away.

Rogers (1967) stresses again and again that when therapists can

communicate to their clients a real and genuine caring, the clients' personalities can develop and become what potentially lies within them to become.

How do you respect yourself? If in a fit of either self-pity or exultation you eat a box of chocolates all at once, do you respect this act, or feel guilty about it? Respecting yourself means that you value yourself as the person you are, with cravings and regrets – and rather than judging yourself, you understand the wonderful diversity of ways of being human. When you can appreciate this in yourself, you can do it more easily with others also.

Trusting

Trusting means having confidence or faith in someone or something. A boat-builder on a desert island would expect to escape unharmed once he or she had built a safe boat. Another person good at gardening or cooking might be more likely to survive on the island by being properly fed. These people would trust themselves and their abilities and skills even under difficult circumstances. What skills and abilities do you have in which you trust? Are there other areas in which you trust in yourself?

In a crisis, many (perhaps most) people lose a certain amount of confidence in themselves. They then need to trust in someone else to help them through such a crisis: a doctor to make a correct diagnosis; a nurse to care competently for them; friends to support them.

As nurses we are constantly in a position to be trusted by our patients. This puts us in a privileged position. It means that we have the patient's confidence even before we do any work with them. In turn, we trust patients and their ability to cope. Our role as nurses is often one of coping, taking over, looking after the helpless, taking responsibility, and acting on behalf of patients who are in need of our particular skills and on which their lives depend. Yet, even in illness and difficulty, patients, like children, are very robust. We need to trust that

they not only can but will cope, whatever that entails. As a
helper you should be sure that you are not

*like the father who 'cares' too much and 'over-protects' his child and
who 'does not trust' the child, and whatever he may think he is doing,
he is responding more to his own needs than to the needs of the child
to grow.* (Mayeroff, 1971, p. 15)

Meize-Grochowski (1984) made a study of the concept of
trust and coined the definition:

*Trust is an attitude bound to time and space in which one relies with
confidence on someone or something. Trust is further characterized by
its fragility.*

In practice, trusting may mean actively giving patients permission to take responsibility for themselves as individuals,
and then encouraging and reinforcing this again and again until
the confidence is there. It also means trusting patients' own
judgement of themselves and their particular situation. For
instance, at some point a patient may refuse to have any more
treatment in the knowledge that there are different ways of
coping with disease that may differ from that of the doctor's
or nurse's expectations. This is not easy to accept as it implies
a rejection of your skills and the care that you have given.
In other words, the fragility (or vulnerability) of both parties
becomes obvious. At such a point you may have to ask, what
is happening here? Is it a *rejection* of *your* skills and available
know-how, or is it an *affirmation* of your client's own person?
If it is the latter, then your skills have actually helped the
client, but perhaps not in the way you had expected. Accepting
a client's decision may indeed be the proof of effective helping.

Caring

*We ultimately feel 'at home' not through dominating or explaining or
appreciating things, but through caring and being cared for.*
(Mayeroff, 1971, p. 54)

The *Oxford English Dictionary* defines 'to care' as meaning to
'feel concern or interest; feel regard, deference, affection'. It
is certainly that, but it is also much more. Caring is 'the human
mode of being', says Roach (1992, p. 2); it is 'humankind at
home, being real, being his- or herself'.

Caring, like its grammatical root-word charity, begins at

home. Caring is not something we do as a duty, or from a sense that if we care, then others will care for us. Caring is so basic that it is that which characterizes us as human beings.

Roach (1992) elaborates her statement by saying that caring is made up of five elements all beginning with the letter 'c': compassion, competence, confidence, conscience and commitment. Compassion is seen as an awareness of a person's relationship with all living creatures. Competence is the knowledge, skill, experience and energy a person brings to professional work with others. Confidence is, according to Roach, the quality that fosters trusting relationships. Conscience is a moral awareness – the compass that directs a person's behaviour – born out of experience and tested in relationships. Commitment is a choice made out of an awareness of desires and obligations.

'We are by nature to be for others', said Roach (1985). When we care for others, then we are also cared for. Mayeroff (1971) goes on:

In a meaningful friendship, caring is mutual, each cares for the other: caring becomes contagious. My caring for the other helps activate his caring for me; and similarly his caring for me helps activate my caring for him, it 'strengthens' me to care for him (p. 26).

Mayeroff (1971) implies that caring qualifies our relationships with one another and that this essentially means 'letting the other grow'. Stories abound of caring having taken place in the most incredible situations, such as battles in the Gulf War and the 'bad old days' of apartheid, and the troubles in Northern Ireland. But perhaps most of us need not look very far before recognizing that caring is instinctual and happens all the time, and simply because we are human.

Caring is mutual; it is reciprocal. When you give, you receive, somehow. But you don't give in order to get. That is the difference between helping – caring – and most other transactions. That is why helping and caring are so satisfying, and so elusive.

Feelings in the helper

The more you know yourself, the more intensely you feel and live, the more 'potent' you become. When you meet with someone in a helping relationship, not only do you feel for and with that other person, that person also arouses feelings in you. Some of these may be good, helpful feelings, and some may be difficult and not easy to deal with.

The following quotation was written about wars and revolutions. It can also apply to nursing.

Confrontation with human pain often creates anger instead of care, irritation instead of sympathy, and even fury instead of compassion. (Nouwen et al, 1982, p. 54)

Strong emotions can be evoked in the face of someone else's suffering. When your emotions are roused in the face of suffering, you may not be able to help. You are too much aware of your own reactive suffering. To be truly human means at times to feel anger, irritation and fury in the face of suffering. Quilliam (1991) has described two nurses who were driven to the point of leaving the profession because unresolved memories were triggered by suffering and they felt hopeless and helpless to do anything about that suffering. Both nurses were helped to release their 'trapped' emotions and see that they do not have to 'care' less but to understand their own feelings better and in context.

Clients may arouse all kinds of feelings in you, from surprise to hope, from irritation to resentment and from helplessness to powerlessness. This is a form of counter-transference (see Chapter 12) and may therefore be misunderstood and misinterpreted. You may have tried every way to be helpful, only to be rejected. Finally you feel resentful at your own inability to cope. If this can be seen and understood as a psychological process rather than a 'fault' or something blameworthy, then it can be dealt with more easily.

You may be left with unfinished business in a helping relationship.

This patient, who was slowly dying, felt helpless in the face of his wife's handling of the domestic affairs and repeated often that he had to knock some sense into her. He is slipping away from me now, and I can't grasp him to knock sense into him. I can only feel the pain of never seeing the result of my help.

You may feel bewildered when patients present problems which you may not understand, or which your moral, ethical or religious beliefs question.

You may be sexually aroused by and attracted to a patient. Or a patient may openly express sexual feelings towards you. This can cause indignation, guilt and annoyance on both sides.

Helping and counselling are based on *feelings*, and on the *person* who has feelings. You are helping that person within a relationship, therefore you are involved, and that means your feelings are important too. This goes right back to awareness, and to starting at home and first looking after yourself. If your own feelings get in the way of helping, then clearly you cannot help effectively. When you know what your feelings are and where they come from and belong, then you will also be able to help others with their feelings and where they come from and belong.

One of the caricatures of helping is the situation where a client says something like 'My whole world collapsed since I broke my arm', and the 'helper' replies, 'You should worry! When I broke my leg. . .'.

To help another person often means that you come across situations that ring bells for you, or touch a raw nerve. They put you in touch with a similar situation or feeling that you have never really 'worked through'. This is particularly common in situations of loss. Your patient only has to mention a parent's recent burial, and you are in touch with what happened to you when you lost one of your parents. There is nothing wrong with that; indeed, if it didn't happen, it would be more alarming. What *is* difficult is if you are then so much 'into' your own feelings that you cannot help, and your client becomes helper to you. And yet, helping *is* reciprocal. You are helped by your client. The crunch is *how* you are helped.

When you know yourself and your feelings, you can use them to help yourself and others. When you do not know them, you will be surprised when they pop up at the most unexpected moments, and then they tend to get out of hand and be destructive. Counselling – and every kind of helping – is for 'better or for worse'. Helping is not just 'doing good', but is a powerful way of being with other people. It is a very satisfying and also a very responsible way of being with others. We should never forget that the first rule of any helping must surely be to *do no harm*.

Beliefs and values

One of the five components of caring is conscience. Like feelings, conscience needs to be known and used in the right way. Like your feelings, your beliefs and values show themselves to others, even though you may not be aware of it.

Ethics is more and more in the public awareness, and rightly so. You need to know where you stand, and from what basis you care and help.

Your personal and professional beliefs and values will therefore colour your work and your relationships with patients, relatives and colleagues. Your attitude will quickly convey itself to all with whom you come in contact. Do you trust a patient, and on what grounds? Do you accept a patient, fleas and all? Do you respect your colleague, even though you consider her overweight, slovenly or lazy? Do your prejudices colour your behaviour?

A patient may be talking with you about fears of dying, and the question of euthanasia comes up. You may have quite strong feelings about it. Do you feel that you have to be helpful, neutral, or to influence this person? How do you know that your views and beliefs are the right ones, or the better ones?

In helping and counselling there is a lot of listening to be done – to yourself and to your clients. Sometimes you may not know what you believe; sometimes you may be very sure. Sometimes you may change completely in the course of a conversation. You may end up by being quite confused about your feelings and your conscience. This is uncomfortable, and quite common. Perhaps you should make friends with your conscience? Helping is not giving the other person your point of view, but enabling others to listen more carefully to their own being and to find the right answer there.

Any situation of change or learning begins with the now, the given. When it comes to self-knowledge, most of us know ourselves very little, perhaps out of fear, perhaps out of neglect.

Helping is not one-sided. It is involved, and involving. You can only help someone out of your own self, your own understanding and from what you have got. It is therefore not only right, but also a duty, to know yourself, to start with yourself and to love yourself. I asked at the beginning whether we can indeed know ourselves. Perhaps yes, perhaps no. What we can do is not to let slip any occasion for knowing ourselves better.

CHAPTER TWO

Support systems

....

Why support is needed

As charity begins at home, so does support. Before we can support others, we need to know that we are supported.

Nurses' need for support is more and more recognized and looked for, though not yet as readily available as might be expected in a 'caring' environment and profession.

Support is needed because nursing and caring by themselves are stressful. Being with and dealing with sick and disabled, frightened and bereaved people all day is stressful, however much a person wants to do this work, enjoys it and is good at it. If we want to be human in our behaviour, then sooner or later we will hurt by what we see and hear. It is also right that we get hurt in this way, because that is how we grow as people and relate to each other as persons. We are not detached bystanders but living beings. Very often it is those who have been hurt and wounded themselves who can relate to patients and clients in a more realistic and empathic way and so help them to adjust or get better more easily and quickly. Just being human is an important aspect of giving care. But this care is costly for the carers. We can count up how much care costs in terms of surgery or medication, but the human cost cannot be counted that easily. Those who are carers do, however, know of the cost to themselves. If this cost is not recognized adequately, resentment creeps in and the care given diminishes.

The causes of stress and inability to care optimally are legion. A few of the more generally acknowledged reasons are: the overall changes taking place in health care; the emphasis on the market place and on economy, efficiency and effectiveness; pressures of education and training and/or uncertainties about them; increasing bureaucracy; limited resources of people and materials; rationalizations; mergers, closures and the changing status of institutions; threats of redundancy; people experiencing themselves to be commodities rather than individuals with feelings, needs and gifts; skill mix; and so on.

To this list, every reader can add her or his own reasons for stress.

This environment and culture contributes greatly to some of the pressures that nurses and carers experience. The work done by Menzies and her subsequent report (Menzies, 1960) highlighted many of the destructive practices that existed in nursing at that time as a 'defence against anxiety'. Much has changed since then, and much has not. 'Defence' is still more often the working model than awareness, and 'attack' tends to be more common than facing the problem.

Daily contact with patients and illness enables nurses to talk easily about issues that are taboo for most people: death, illness, facing diminishment, decisions on who and how to treat, and dealing with mental illness, to mention just a few. To go with a person into these realms is like constantly overstepping conventionally accepted boundaries; this cannot be done without cost.

The combination of emotional giving and pressures from many sides is a potent force which may push nurses to the brink and cause them to become disillusioned, cut corners, use and abuse each other, become hard and uncaring, and burn out. The last straw for many is when they cannot challenge wrong-doing for fear that they might be called trouble-makers. How far can you go before compromising your integrity?

On the whole, nurses are not particularly kind, generous and supportive of each other. It is astonishing how we can be regarded as 'angels' by patients but often act like 'devils' to colleagues. The nursing culture is still one in which the stiff upper lip is preferred to the soft underbelly. It is perhaps not surprising therefore that many means of support are still theoretical rather than practical. It is not until the culture becomes caring – as the work done in it is caring – that the need for support and the giving of support become essential.

Staff support

In its publication *A Charter for Staff Support* the National Association for Staff Support (NASS, 1992) makes many valuable statements about the need for staff support and policy principles, and the rights and responsibilities of receivers and givers of support. At the beginning of the Charter are six points describing what staff support is:

Staff support involves more than incorporating recognized support systems, or bringing in a service at a time of crisis. Although these things are very important, staff support also involves the creation of

a caring and healthy working environment and culture, which is an integral part of every institutional setting.
It ensures that a variety of support mechanisms are available.
It assists individuals to recognize stressful situations and to be aware of their own responses to stress and recognize their limitations.
It enables staff carers to acknowledge sensitivity and to develop and use their own coping mechanisms and strengths.
It turns supervision into a recreative process which encourages, teaches and improves the quality of professional work.
It fosters a management structure that ensures individuals are valued.

These points constitute a philosophical basis for staff support on which the practical implications can be built. The emphasis is on encouragement, empowerment and enthusiasm, in contrast to the way in which support is viewed by many people: as a last resort for someone who has failed. Staff support is *a good thing*, not a stick with which to beat failures into submission.

The support systems available

There are many possibilities of, and for, support. The first few mentioned are classic examples.

Counsellors

A counsellor for the staff, and for nurses in particular, can be a most valuable support. This is for several reasons: a counsellor can give clients the safety to explore their real feelings, and the permission to talk about things that are of the utmost importance to them, particularly the knowledge that they have been heard (Crawley, 1983). Most problems presented to a counsellor concern a relationship – with a colleague, manager, patient, relative or immediate family – and it is therefore important that the issues be discussed in a relationship.

So that there is indeed 'safety' for a client, a counsellor needs to be completely independent, i.e. not attached to a school or college of nursing, or to administration, either in salary or in the location of the office. A study by Doust (1991) among student nurses using counselling services found that 90% of them 'had a positive attitude to the service' but they still had anxieties about approaching it: 'The more students believed that (any) information might get passed on, the more negatively they felt towards the counselling service'. Davies (1993) found that 93% of the respondents to a questionnaire at a health centre indicated that they would return for counselling if they needed further help. Most of the people surveyed were seen between four and six times only. Perhaps the initial step to counselling remains difficult, but, once discovered, counselling becomes not only a help but also a tool for learning to cope on one's own.

Groups

The next important area of support is groups. Most people need to talk to other people in order to feel appreciated. Seeing that others have the same needs and problems is invaluable, and this cannot be learnt in isolation, hence the need for a group.

Such support groups for nurses can deal with issues related particularly to individual and personal management skills, professional identity, techniques for stress management, methods of conflict management, personal relationships and how to increase staff members' sense of self-esteem and self-confidence.

To be effective, support for nurses needs to be continuous, and groups are the most perennial form of giving support; they are flexible in time, context, content and style. But support groups will function well only if they have an aim. This is normally awareness and action, but may also be orientation to a specific goal, although this may be a changeable goal. A group that meets solely for the sake of meeting may not be successful, unless that is its specific goal. Groups may be used for a limited period only, or may persist. The membership may change, but any changes should be discussed and implemented, not just allowed to happen, otherwise the group will disintegrate.

Bailey *et al.* (1994) described an educational support group for a cohort of RMN (Registered Mental Nurse) students and two of their teachers. The group had the double task of learning experientially about group theory and practice, and providing support for its members in their educational endeavours. The group stayed together for about a year, and their evaluation showed that they had moved through all the classical stages of theory, had formed strong peer relationships and that communication was better between students and teachers. Their article describes the theory of group work well. It is also an interesting account of a group formed for a specific task. Not all groups function best under the pressure of self-evaluation, but the pressure thus created also increases the conscious learning.

Occupational health service (OHS)

Seen as part of an overall supportive environment, staff in the OHS can advise employees on how to improve and maintain health, or prevent the occurrence of ill-health or injury.

Occupational health is increasingly of interest to employers because the costs of 'sickness absence, staff turnover and recruitment, low morale and decreased productivity' (Marks and Hingley, 1991) are beginning to be counted and felt. In a climate of reduced and restricted resources, the cost in terms of human suffering is moving management to do something. Staff in the OHS and similar services in industry are encouraged as front-line workers to rectify the losses.

Many problems become large because no one is available to listen. Once the problem has been heard and shared, it is often halved in magnitude. The OHS is one possible setting for lending an ear.

Owen (1993) produces a yearly literature review on 'Stress, Coping Mechanisms and Support Systems for Professional Carers' which describes new directions, developments and achievements in these fields of support. This and other material on stress and support is available from the National Association for Staff Support (see address at the end of this chapter).

Education and teaching

A strong area of support for nurses is education and teaching. Nurses need to be skilled not only in nursing activities, but also in the human activities of communicating, relating and managing. Learning about counselling should not simply be a matter of buying a book; it should also include teaching in the health care environment.

Systematic education should include such topics as stress and its management; self-awareness; personal and professional ethics, with particular reference to any specialty in which the nurses are working; supportive and interpersonal skills, such as helping and counselling; and leadership skills. When nurses are skilled in these areas, then they can give optimum care.

At a conference organized by the Health Education Authority in January 1994 (*Nursing Standard*, 1994), designed to improve the lives of the NHS workforce, the head of the NHS Management Executive told delegates that 'there is a compelling moral, legal and economic case for pursuing vigorously' an initiative to help stressed health care staff to cope with their work. It is perhaps a sad reflection on our time that only when something has a 'value for money' stamp on it will it be taken seriously. With staff being the most valuable asset an employer has, surely stress management should be available to all health care personnel.

Self-awareness is not something that can be taught easily, but people trained in interactive skills may be able to teach the subject in workshop format (Tschudin, 1991) or as part of studies in human behaviour, psychology or sociology. Buckroyd and Smith (1990) have described a course at a university for training experienced nurses in their counselling role. They found that they had to help nurses to examine their own feelings and underlying psychological issues of helping before they could be effective counsellors. Their conclusion was that

a holistic approach to the needs of patients and nurses be taught from the start of training; feelings are not an optional extra. . . We urge the importance of recognition and respect for feelings in health service organisations. Carers should not have to take a course at an external institution to explore emotional issues; that should be an integral part of the work. (Buckroyd and Smith, 1990)

Personal and professional ethics is becoming ever more important. The emphasis on the market place in health care rests on the idea of personal choice and therefore personal autonomy to choose. This can be a difficult notion for patients and clients to accept and for nurses and carers to put into practice. The difference here between giving advice, information and counselling is of prime importance. Nurses need therefore to have a good grounding in some basic ethical principles and language, but they must also be able to reason morally. Awareness of and training in values and value-clarification (Tschudin, 1992) is as important as ethics (Tschudin and Marks-Maran, 1993).

The acquisition of supportive and interpersonal skills is essential for anyone who has to deal with people. Nurses, who usually meet people at crisis points in their lives, need to have not only communication skills, but also a good knowledge of the psychological needs of people in various situations. Macleod Clark and colleagues (1991) have devised a hierarchy of activities in the form of a pyramid, of progression from communication to counselling skills:

At the base lie communication skills, which are the foundation for all interpersonal relationships, and are used most widely in the caring professions. With further training and self-awareness, counselling skills can be built on to communication skills, forming the next layer up. Counselling, which requires special training and particular skills, lies at the top of the pyramid.

This shows that increased training leads to increased expertise.

Reflective practice is now a well-used tool for learning, and the use of actual examples by students and participants in further training programmes is seen to be as effective as role play and other teaching methods. Both 'reflection-in-action and reflection-on-action' (Schön, 1987) foster awareness and skills.

Supervision

Supportive and competent supervision is essential if nurses are to give their best to the care of the ill, frail and vulnerable (Ogier and Cameron-Buccheri, 1990). Yet most nurses have no experience of supervision and therefore do not know what it *is*. Broadly speaking, supervision can be described as having three main functions:

1. A management function.
2. A support function.
3. A training and staff development function.

Fox (1994), writing about clinical supervision, lists four topics that can be recognized:

1. Maintenance of professional standards.
2. The supervisor acts as role model.
3. Supervision reduces stress.
4. Supervision provides education and training.

There emerges, therefore, a composite role 'for the clinical supervisor beyond that of manager, mentor or preceptor' (Fox, 1994).

It may be useful, given the context of this book, to be clear about the kind of supervision that is meant here. Clinical supervision could and should apply to all nurses for their practical care. Those nurses who have a counselling role or who deliberately use counselling as part of their care should also have supervision for this work. The British Association for Counselling (BAC) (1994a) has described this as 'regular and appropriate supervision/consultative support'. It may be possible to combine the clinical and counselling aspects in supervision; indeed, this might be the ideal. It is also possible that these aspects cannot be combined – due to inexperience of the supervisor in one or other subject – and that a nurse may therefore need two supervisors. As long as the role of each is clear, no difficulty should arise.

Supervision gives rights and responsibilities to both parties. The supervisor should ensure that the supervisee is aware of policies, has an adequate workload, has the tools available to carry out the work; that the work is fairly evaluated and this is communicated to the supervisee; and that the supervisee is supported, particularly during stressful times.

The supervisee on the other hand is accountable to the supervisor for the work done and the way it is carried out.

Both parties are responsible for seeing that supervision takes place on a regular basis. Together they should determine the supervisee's developmental needs, and both should agree how these will be met.

Heywood Jones (1989) tells of a health visitor with considerable experience who also showed enthusiasm and innovative practice in a new post. Her difficulty was that she did not keep her secondary records up to date. She was aware of this and had asked for help by requesting her manager to ask for the records on a regular basis. This help was not forthcoming and the health visitor was finally brought before a professional conduct committee, accused of fifteen charges concerning documentation.

This incident illustrates several factors:

a) The pressure of work.
b) The pressure of documentation.
c) The pressure to be innovative.
d) Lack of supervision.
e) Lack of personal support (she knew her weak spot but was not helped to change).
f) The inability to deal with the problem in a supportive way, using punishment instead.

On a practical level, Ogier and Cameron-Buccheri (1990) found that supervision was more satisfactory when it was supportive rather than controlling. This meant mainly asking open questions such as 'How are you getting on in this area?' rather than checking: 'Have you done. . . ?'

Sometimes there is a need to talk to someone about a particular patient, but it is impossible to do so to a colleague or a senior member of the team because of issues of confidentiality. A supervisor is then not only the ideal but also the appropriate person. Jacobs (1982, p. 37) suggested that *particular anxieties which many counsellors have are about handling feelings of love, aggression, sexuality and power. Training for (pastoral) counselling requires some mastery of the anxiety about such feelings, whether they are shown by clients, or are seen in different forms in counsellors themselves.*

These are not issues that can be solved in a few minutes, and cannot be talked about to just anybody. Therefore supervision that is ongoing, supportive and challenging is essential.

Who should be a supervisor is an essential question. Ideally it should be a person of experience who has insight into the supervisee's work. This may be another nurse or another health professional. In the case of a supervisor for counselling, this should not be a person from the same unit or department as the supervisee.

Some supervision is possible in groups, either outside the working environment or in a support group. The support given by a whole team to a particular patient may be discussed, and different styles and approaches examined. The issue of confidentiality is, however, a delicate one in groups and needs constantly to be kept in mind and respected.

Groups can be very useful, and indeed powerful, sources of supervision. Forms of self-sharing by all the members of the group can lead them to see where the wider issues in dealings with clients might be improved.

Fox (1994) has also outlined some of the difficulties with supervision. Clinical supervision is most effective when there is a long-term relationship between supervisor and supervisee, but given the economic climate and short-term contracts, such relationships are becoming rare. With more care taking place in the community, there is a geographical problem of distances for effective supervision and meeting. The availability for clinical supervision is decreased in the context of skill mix. The increasing use of 12-hour shifts leaves little time for overlap and supervision and educational support.

The papers by Kohner (1994) and Butterworth and Faugier (1994) have made the idea of clinical supervision one of urgent debate. Like everything else, viewed in one light, clinical supervision is a good thing, but it can also be abused.

Who should choose the person who is going to carry out the review? Should individual nurses be allowed to choose their own supervisors? What if there is a conflict of interest between clinical care and institutional management goals? Who should set the standards for clinical supervision? (Castledine, 1994)

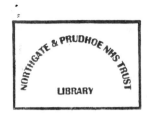

These real difficulties should not, however, scupper the concept of supervision and the real need for it. They may simply mean that all possibilities for staff care should be taken seriously and constantly reviewed.

Other forms of support

There are various other forms of support available and possible in institutions and health care settings. One such is 'time out' arrangements. This often means a given amount of time being available to nurses – perhaps an hour a week to do with as they please, but such time should be considered as support, not simply free time. Thus, one person might use it for supervision, another to go swimming and yet another might do some studying. It might be possible to review these arrangements during supervision and see that they are used in the most appropriate and helpful way.

Professional organizations and unions usually deal with work-related issues. These are important elements to promote and maintain a healthy and safe working environment.

Chaplaincy services usually offer support to patients and staff alike. Some services are more willing and better staffed than others and it is therefore a question of finding and trying the service. As with other possible services, such as social services or specialist nurses, personal contact and availability are perhaps the biggest influences on their use.

A sense of personal responsibility for shaping and creating a caring environment is seen to be as important as the more formal support systems in the *Charter for Staff Support* (NASS, 1992). Some of the ways in which this can be carried out are:

a) Recognizing the effects of stress on self and colleagues.
b) Offering personal support and encouragement to colleagues.
c) Offering thanks and appreciation where appropriate.
d) Considering ways in which one's own environment can be improved.
e) Knowing exactly what local facilities are available.
f) Knowing what one's own professional organization can do to help.
g) Knowing the arrangements for reporting failure to provide basic individual rights.

The counselling role of senior personnel

Most nurses have some reference in their contract to counselling colleagues and personnel for whom they are responsible. This is potentially a grey area because the word 'counselling' is often misused in such settings. Counselling is understood to be a helping process (see Chapter 3), but when used by a senior with a junior employee what is generally meant is a disciplinary procedure, and the word 'counselling' gives a false impression and false expectations. Both types of intervention have their place, but it should be clear to both parties which type is used in which circumstances. A short overview of the *counselling* role of three types of senior personnel follows, which outlines the function rather than the techniques used in such circumstances.

Tutor–counsellors

Nurses who adopt a combined tutor–counsellor role may find themselves faced with multiple moral dilemmas arising from their contact with learners. Can they keep faith with their responsibility of providing information to the nursing school or administration, and yet keep a total counselling commitment of confidence to nurse learners? (Bailey, 1981)

As soon as counselling is done by people who are in a hierarchical relationship to each other, the dynamics of counselling change. Confidentiality, documentation and referral become immediately obvious issues.

On entry into nursing, a young person is allocated to a tutor who has that student's welfare particularly in mind. There may be other such 'special' people for the new student, such as a mentor or other senior nurses. These people are then not only their teachers, but take on a role of parent or someone who is 'sorting out my life' (Doust, 1991). For some students, especially very young people, this may be ideal, but for others it may cause confusion. When a problem arises, they feel obliged to go to their tutor who they may respect as a teacher but would not like to pour their heart out to. Where else are they to go?

A sensitive tutor is aware of these possible pitfalls, and in many schools of nursing and campuses systems are in operation where students choose the tutors they relate to most easily, rather than the other way round.

Nevertheless, the issue remains how far students can take a personal problem to a tutor without it interfering with their academic career. When does a personal problem become a career problem, or vice versa? For this and other such reasons it is imperative that teachers and tutors have a good grounding in counselling skills.

Manager–counsellors

Manager–counsellors encounter similar pitfalls as teachers and tutors, except that they deal with qualified staff, not students.

Are managers really able to counsel, or are they inevitably and by necessity disciplining? The junior member in the hierarchy, when called to see the line manager, may be suspicious, particularly if it is not made clear from the outset what the agenda is. This has been graphically described by Burnard (1990a), who writes of being

reassured by a ward sister that a student (whom) she was finding difficult would no longer be so. She said to me: 'Don't worry, Mr Burnard, I've given her a bloody good counselling!'

Nurses may feel that this is not counselling as such, but more like an appraisal, whereby they are encouraged to change their attitudes and behaviour and to think things out for themselves, so long as they come to the conclusions desired by the counsellor.

Managers have to manage, and disciplining is part of this function. It is easy then to say that they are 'counselling', because it sounds less severe. The fact is that neither party is helped by such deception because discipline still has to be upheld, and counselling did not happen.

Hore (1984) defined managers as people who must achieve results through others, and counselling as a non-directive process that helps people to help themselves. These two approaches to people essentially complement each other. When, therefore, manager–counsellors have objectives other than those of the organization or of education, they embark on the slippery slope to manipulation, which can be a seductive trap for some managers.

When managers can make it clear to their staff which of the two approaches is being used, then clarity will be not only maintained, but fostered, and both sides will benefit.

However, it is almost impossible for a manager in an interview to say 'Now I am managing' (i.e. concerned with the organization) or 'Now I am counselling' (i.e. helping the client to help herself or himself). A good manager, though, who has some counselling skills, will always concentrate on the person rather than the problem.

The aim is not to solve one particular problem but to assist the individual to grow, *so that he can cope with the present problem and with later problems in a better integrated fashion.* (Rogers, 1978, p. 6)

More and more organizations realize that their staff function better when encouraged to take part in decisions and when these decisions are then tried and implemented. When empowerment is not just a politically correct expression but a reality, then the manager–counsellors will be using counselling skills to help the workforce to help themselves and managerial skills to get the best for the organization. Then they are really empowering others – and themselves into the bargain.

Colleague counsellors

Most of the helping done by colleagues happens at points of crisis. It is impossible to be alongside pain and suffering all day without being affected by it. Much of the care given is at great personal cost. 'You see them when the patient keeps ringing the bell and they grimace to themselves. Then they go up to the patient all smiles' (Smith, 1989). At some stage, a breaking point is reached and the lid comes off. The first to catch what is coming out may be a colleague. Helping each other in such situations is not only necessary, but often very beneficial for relationships all round.

But can this be continued in the long term? And officially? Counselling colleagues can lead into conflicts of loyalties. Are nurses firstly loyal to 'the hospital (which employs them), the physician (with whom they work), the client (for whom they provide care), or the nursing profession (to which they belong)?' (Benjamin and Curtis, 1986, p. 23). Loyalty to colleagues has always been highly prized, which is perhaps why much helping goes on among colleagues, and little independent help is either sought or used. When you are helping colleagues you may have to consider their and your ethical standpoints. 'Loyalty' has sometimes been blamed for blatant disregard of major issues. Nurses may not be given realistic help because colleagues have covered up. This is precisely where counselling colleagues can turn into a curse what was meant to be a blessing. Such helping needs to go on, but with eyes wide open and with as much clarity and empathy as can be mustered.

The increasing incidence of drug and alcohol abuse among nurses has often been highlighted (Booth, 1985). The sheer availability of drugs makes nurses vulnerable to abuse, although Booth claims that 'most of the factors influencing alcohol and drug consumption by nurses are unrelated to the nursing profession'. This is significant, because it shows that nurses still take on a persona when they put on their uniform and almost deny that they have another life; and also that nurses have cared very little for each other as *persons*.

Burnard (1990b) writes of the situation of a nurse manager going to a colleague in a more junior position for help and counselling. With a less strong sense of hierarchy having to be maintained at work, positions get blurred, and with them also the traditional boundaries. Yet 'it may be easier for a person in a senior position to talk (more) readily about his problem than it may be for someone junior to adopt the role of counsellor'. Once the culture of the hierarchy has been instilled it is very difficult to remove it again. So the person who is junior may always feel inferior, even though she or he may be many years older than the boss.

When a senior chooses a junior for help there may be many reasons: her or his age, experience, reputation (as a listener), 'safety' in the sense that she or he may not have any ambitions to defend, or is known not to talk 'shop'. Whatever the reasons, it is not easy for the helper to be put into this position. But compassion and duty oblige her or him to stay there and help in the best way possible. The skills used are the same; the process is the same. What may be different in this situation are the boundaries: what they are, where they are, and what they may mean. Perhaps knowing one's personal boundaries is a first step – and yet one more reason for self-awareness and self-knowledge. This also means that loyalty to oneself and one's values and instincts should perhaps be added to the loyalties described above.

Which support should you have?

Because of the various pressures under which nurses work, support could be seen as yet one more thing to do or go to. Or a manager might say that you can have support, but you have to choose one from a range of possibilities. The different areas outlined above do not in any way constitute all the possibilities. Nurses who have felt strongly enough that they need support have used all manner of ways to get it. They meet in the pub at lunchtime once a fortnight; they meet in each other's houses; they ask a social worker or chaplain to supervise a few of them in a group; they use friends as counsellors; they pass books and articles around on specific topics of mutual interest. Some area health authorities have funded innovative projects where counselling is available within a setting of advice and information. There are peripatetic counsellors. Others have set up help-lines for colleagues in similar work.

Support is more and more seen to be something comprehensive rather than just one thing, and something that is part of the whole ethos of caring. Support systems should exist in many forms and one person should have access to as many such forms as possible. Different types will suit different people at different situations and times.

On the whole it is helpful to have a specific person who acts as a support in the first instance, and also to have one or more groups who give support in different ways. It may be useful to ask yourself who you might telephone at 3 a.m. when you have a particular problem which cannot wait until the morning? Who is the person you trust to support you then? You may never need to phone this person, but simply to know who it is may be the most important support you have. Such a person is *for* you in every kind of way.

Accessing support

In most nursing situations, a direct line manager is still usually considered to be the automatic supervisor, that is, teachers and tutors for student nurses, ward managers for ward staff, and senior nurses for ward and community managers. For most practical reasons this is perfectly normal and adequate, and also helpful. In some instances, though, especially when confidentiality is at stake, the immediate superior is not necessarily the best person to turn to. It is then that it matters who the person is who supports you most or best. In situations of real need you should not be made to feel guilty for not going through the 'proper channels'. In case of any come-back or repercussions of such actions, the important thing is to be able to give a reason for having acted in the way you did. Reporting back later to the immediate superior may be a good gesture.

Perhaps there are support groups available and you do not know whether to join one, or which one. Talking with the leader of such a group may indicate whether it is possible to join such a group or not. It is not easy to try out groups, as this can cause disruption. If you know some of the people in a group, it will be easier to join.

If you feel unable to join an existing group, it is always possible to form a group yourself with friends or colleagues. Some basic knowledge of group dynamics is necessary if the group is formal. Even informal groups function better when there are just one or two rules observed. The literature which NASS has produced may be helpful here.

In a newsletter produced by the NASS (1994), Christine Hancock, General Secretary of the Royal College of Nursing, writes:

The NHS is well known for shooting its messengers and punishing its whistleblowers. This situation must be addressed urgently. In future, asking for support or for advice must not be seen as evidence of an inability to cope, but as a primary step in disaster prevention and an essential component of quality assurance.

Accessing supervision or counselling may be more difficult because it demands a commitment. These forms of support are ongoing and can be quite intensive. The skills needed here are:

a)   Deciding what it is you are looking for.
b)   Negotiating with the supervisor/counsellor for what you need in terms of numbers of (initial) meetings, length of each meeting, what it costs (if anything), and any work to be done between meetings.
c)   Ensuring that the supervisor/counsellor is competent (and suitably qualified) in her or his field. (The British Association for Counselling recommends that those who call themselves 'counsellors' should have had 450 hours of training.)

It should not be impertinent to ask the potential counsellor whether she or he is qualified. If a person is trained, there is nothing to hide; if not, you can still decide to be supervised or counselled, depending on your judgement of the person.

Perhaps the most important skill in looking for support and supervision is knowing and recognizing one's limits and boundaries (Faugier, 1991; Speck, 1992). To acknowledge that a situation is too difficult is not necessarily to admit defeat, but to be realistic. Equally, to know where a boundary lies means being able to go as far as the boundary, and perhaps push it out further with experience. Not to know a boundary often means not being able to go as far as may be possible, for fear of losing control. Helping skills grow with experience, and it is unrealistic to think that simply by putting on a uniform we should be able to help the world. We can do damage to other people by inexperience, but we can also do damage by pride. Somewhere between these extremes lies the middle ground of being confident of one's ability and the courage to stand by someone even when the going is tough.

Only nurses who are supported can give optimal care. We cannot give and give and empty ourselves in the service of others without being damaged. I sometimes have an image of nurses being like wine boxes: very useful inventions, holding a lot of liquid which can be used or drained slowly. But in the end you are left with a collapsed bag and an open tap – no good to anyone. The secret is how to stay full and useful, able to give and able to receive. Both these elements have to be learned and practised.

National Association for Staff Support (NASS)
9 Caradon Close
Woking GU21 3DU.

CHAPTER THREE

Counselling and counselling skills

....

What is counselling?

What is counselling? This question must have been asked by everyone who has ever tried to help another person. Or perhaps more specifically, the question might be, 'Am I just helping or am I counselling?'

A dictionary will probably define counselling as giving counsel or advice, or making recommendations. This is considered by those who counsel as an inadequate definition, and even contrary to their practice.

Nurse (1978) cites some early definitions, among them one by J.H. Wallis: counselling is 'a dialogue in which one person helps another who has some difficulty that is important to him'.

The British Association for Counselling (BAC) has frequently rewritten its definition. The *Code of Ethics and Practice for Counsellors* (1993) describes 'The Nature of Counselling' in the following way:

The overall aim of counselling is to provide an opportunity for the client to work towards living in a more satisfying and resourceful way. The term 'counselling' includes work with individuals, pairs or groups of people, often, but not always, referred to as 'clients'. The objectives of particular counselling relationships will vary according to the client's needs. Counselling may be concerned with developmental issues, addressing and resolving specific problems, making decisions, coping with crisis, developing insight and knowledge, working through feelings of inner conflict or improving relationships with others. The counsellor's role is to facilitate the client's work in ways which respect the client's values, personal resources and capacity for self-determination.

Only when both the user and the recipient explicitly agree to enter into a counselling relationship does it become 'counselling' rather than the use of 'counselling skills'.

It is not possible to make a generally accepted distinction between counselling and psychotherapy. There are well founded traditions which use the terms interchangeably and others which distinguish them. Regardless of the theoretical approaches preferred by individual counsellors, there are ethical issues which are common to all counselling situations.

The *Code of Ethics and Practice for Counselling Skills* (1989) of the BAC states that:

The term 'counselling skills' does not have a single definition which is universally accepted. For the purpose of this code, 'counselling skills' are distinguished from 'listening skills' and from 'counselling'. Although the distinction is not always a clear one, because the term 'counselling skills' contains elements of these other two activities, it has its own place in the continuum between them. What distinguishes the use of counselling skills from these other activities are the intentions of the user, which is to enhance the performance of their functional role, as line manager, nurse, tutor, social worker, personnel officer, voluntary worker etc. The recipient will, in turn, perceive them in that role.

Ask yourself the following questions:

a) Are you using counselling skills to enhance your communication with someone but without taking on the role of their counsellor?
b) Does the recipient perceive you as acting within your professional/caring role (which is NOT that of being their counsellor)?

>   *(i)   If the answer is YES to both of these questions, you are using counselling skills in your functional role.*
>   *(ii)   If the answer is NO to both, you are counselling.*
>   *(iii) If the answer is YES to one and NO to the other, you have a conflict of expectations and should resolve it.*

Only when both the user and recipient explicitly contract to enter into a counselling relationship does it cease to be 'using counselling skills' and becomes 'counselling'.

The significant difference between 'counselling' and 'using counselling skills' is a contract. This can be anything from a signed document to the most simple of verbal agreements. This will be dealt with in more detail in Chapter 12.

This book concentrates on counselling skills, but this is not possible without also looking at counselling as such. Where appropriate, the difference will be highlighted. But whether counselling, or using counselling skills, there are some basic elements that are common to both situations. These are discussed in this chapter.

The relationship

Any helping, be this by counselling or supervision, caring for old or young, sick or well, needs two (or more) people: the client and the helper. But the third element is the relationship they establish and this is most important.

These three elements (the patient or client, the helper and the relationship between them) have to be studied, understood, supported and constantly evaluated. Caring is not a one-way process, nor even a two-way one. It is a dynamic, circular or spiral process in which one element influences the other two, and they may never have quite the same influence twice.

In nursing we pay much attention to the patient or client, and rightly so. We pay much less attention to helpers and their needs, and until recently we have almost neglected the relationship. By learning interpersonal skills, assertiveness and relaxation techniques, nurses are taking themselves more seriously as people and as professionals. However, so far it has rarely been accepted that patients really get better more quickly and more completely when they are cared for by nurses with whom they get on.

The following quote was written for counsellors, but the word 'counsellor' can easily be substituted with 'helper' here:

If I can create a relationship characterized on my part
    by a genuineness and transparency, in which I am my real feelings
    by a warm acceptance of and prizing of the other person as a separate individual
    by a sensitive ability to see his world and himself as he sees them
Then the other individual in the relationship
    will experience and understand aspects of himself which previously he has repressed
    will find himself becoming better integrated, more able to function effectively
    will become more similar to the person he would like to be
    will be more self-directing and self-confident
    will become more of a person, more unique and more self-expressive
    will be more understanding, more acceptant of others
    will be able to cope with the problems of life more adequately and more comfortably.

(Rogers, 1961, p. 37)

What Rogers is saying, and what the various definitions point to, is that the skills used in counselling are almost incidental. What matters is how the two people relate to each other. The skills of counselling *are* important, but that 'something other' – those indefinable 'vibes' – are just as important.

Skills

Counselling skills are a specific type of communication skill which some people use with expertise. They are used entirely for the purpose of helping one person at one time, or several together in a group or family, to live 'in a more satisfying and resourceful way' (BAC, 1993). These skills can be used in a short interaction or a long-term relationship. The only crucial thing is that the skills are used.

The process

For helping and caring effectively four steps are necessary:

1. To define the starting point and clarify the problem.
2. To gain some insight into why there is a problem.
3. To discover a goal to aim for.
4. To explore the ways and means of getting there.

Helping and counselling are goal oriented and are not simply used to analyse a problem. But counselling is not *problem* oriented either. It is *person* oriented, that is, the person-with-the-problem is helped. This means a flow, or movement forward, from one point to another; from problem to goal; from dissatisfaction to satisfaction; and from being 'stuck' to resourcefulness. For this to take place there has to be a relationship with at least one other person.

Self-help

A situation in which counselling skills are used is not 'doing for' the other. Counselling, and this sort of helping, does not prescribe. Counselling enables the client not only to solve a problem, but to be a more effective person, and that means knowing how to be effective. Self-help, or empowerment, are the outcomes of helping and counselling. This presupposes that 'when we treat people with the expectation that they will conduct themselves as healthy, attentive individuals, they generally do so' (Goldman and Morrison, 1984).

What counselling is not

It is easier to say what counselling is *not* than to say what it is. Giving advice, giving information, coaching, disciplinary interviews, guidance, recommending, persuading, instructing and analysing are *not* counselling. Any of these activities may, however, lead to counselling.

The word counselling has crept into situations which are far from what the word means to a professional counsellor. 'I had to counsel her' is a remark which points more to probable difficulties with interpersonal skills by a manager than to a client's implied misdemeanour.

Nurses often have to give information, advice and guidance. They often have to instruct patients and colleagues in the use of equipment or techniques. They also often use counselling skills. One of those skills is to clarify issues, situations and relationships that are, or present, problems. By also being clear about what the method of helping is – giving information, advice or guidance, or using counselling skills to facilitate the client's work – the whole thing becomes easier. There is a sense in which 'calling a spade a spade' is truly helpful; both parties know where they stand with each other.

Giving advice, information or coaching is no less important, but by calling them 'counselling' they are not made more important. Each in its place could not be replaced by the other.

When should it be 'counselling'?

Most nurses use counselling skills frequently with clients, most often in one-off situations. This is therefore short-term work and usually relates to a single issue. Out of this can, and sometimes do, come more contacts and more exploration. It is often the case that when one aspect of a person is examined and better understood, then other issues present themselves, also begging to be understood. Thus a counselling situation arises which might need more expert help, and this implies a contract, even if it is only 'I'll be back tomorrow and we can then talk further'.

From an opening remark it is often possible to judge whether the person is looking for someone with counselling skills to help, or is needing counselling. The following statements point to the need for a response from someone with counselling skills:

I just want to have a cry (get angry, feel afraid). . .
I need someone to listen to me. . .
I want to clear up the confusion about. . .
I don't know what's going on but I don't feel right. . .
I just can't make up my mind. . .
I want to help her, but I don't seem to get it right. . .

The following remarks might need help with counselling:

I need someone to help me through. . .
I want to understand. . .
I need to explore. . .
I want to feel differently about. . .

I need to change. . .

Helping someone effectively means picking up such opening remarks and following them through. Anyone who is in a situation, physically, mentally and spiritually, where he or she would rather not be, needs help. Very often it is difficult to know what the situation or problem actually is. It may be a practical problem, but if individuals are unable to solve a practical problem then they experience difficulties with the feelings involved, the mindsets, or personal abilities and inabilities encountered. This is when another person helps by being alongside with counselling skills. Such skills either help the person to be supported, help an individual to gain insight, or enable someone to change an attitude. If this skilled helping is done within the framework of nursing or caring generally, then clearly it is counselling – but from within the functional role of a nurse or helper. Any such situation can lead to further helping and counselling and this should be kept in mind and followed up if necessary.

For whom is counselling suitable?

The times and situations when counselling or the use of counselling skills are unsuitable are probably few. People with learning difficulties are possibly not helped by counselling as such, although they need a great deal of care and attention. On the other hand, people with mental illness need a great deal of counselling. The type of help given is then more specific to the person's illness, and may also be given with clear guidelines and often on a one-to-one basis, but also in groups.

People with undiagnosed mental illness may possibly not be helped. This may be difficult to spot and nurses may feel that they have failed a person. When a patient's symptoms worsen or existing symptoms develop (Clarke, 1986), it is likely that counselling has reached its limits and that some other or more therapeutic help is needed.

Counselling may also be an inappropriate form of help for some people whose culture or religion deals with personal problems in ways that are different from those of recognized counselling patterns.

In addition to those with a recognized psychiatric illness or people with learning difficulties, most people can at times benefit from counselling. The psychologist Sigmund Freud believed that people near or above the age of 50 years are not educable and that psychotherapy is not possible with them (Scrutton, 1989, p. 19). The 'theory he evolved was influenced by preconceptions, derived from the physical sciences, that had little to do with actual people' (Lomas, 1994, p. 52). This may be just as well as otherwise a good many of us might be beyond the pale!

That children need counselling just as much as adults is also being increasingly acknowledged. Counselling in this field is necessarily specialized and adapted to the world and understanding of children, although the basic concepts and theories still apply.

In your work as a nurse you will find many opportunities for using counselling skills and counselling as such. It is often in unexpected situations that help is most needed and most welcome: the patients who seem to cope well, but might just drop a hint that there is 'a little difficulty at home'; the person who had a colostomy and, on asking if his or her sex life is going to be alright, is told by the surgeon that there should be no problem, but who subsequently reveals to the nurse that he or she is homosexual (Wells, 1988, p. 466); or the mother of a young baby who tells the health visitor that she thinks that her teenage step-daughter is taking drugs. These are unexpected situations, and perhaps one of the qualities that nurses have to develop is a certain unshockability. More frequently, perhaps, the patient's problems are less unusual; or the nurse sees by the patient's behaviour or body language that there is something amiss.

Most help given by nurses starts with a crisis, often of an emotional kind. The use of counselling skills then lays the ground for more in-depth work and developmental counselling. Once the immediate need for help is over, the person can begin to change. This may be difficult to achieve in the nursing setting, when patients are seldom cared for on a long-term basis. The ideal setting may be in the community, in rehabilitation areas, or in any situation of long-term care where patients must often make considerable adaptations in their attitudes to health and illness.

It can be very helpful to know our limits and to be clear what kind of help we can offer in what circumstances. It is unrealistic to think that counselling solves every problem; indeed, it is not meant to do this. The use of counselling skills is, however, not limited. All those in the caring professions should have some of these skills. We are not born with them, although some people are naturally more empathic than others; but we can all improve our ways of helping – and in the process improve our understanding of ourselves, usually to good effect.

CHAPTER FOUR

Models for counselling

....

Why have models for helping?

It has often been said that all you need to do to help another person is listen. That is correct up to a point. If you then know how to listen and what to listen for, you will listen better.

Imagine that your client – colleague or patient – makes a statement to you, 'I just can't go on like this any longer'. This implies that your client is emotionally and perhaps also physically, in a state where she or he would rather not be. If you simply listened, you would not answer. This could be a sign of your pity and sympathy; of your helplessness in the face of suffering; or your inability to cope with a difficult situation. Your silence may be interpreted very differently depending on the body language of both of you, on the relationship which you have and on the tone of voice in which the statement was said – whether it implied defeat or anger. Listening, therefore, is not simply sitting with another person and soaking up what is said. Listening implies responding. *How* you respond is a skill: the counselling skill. The client may perceive this as interaction and help, but not as special expertise. Depending on your skills, you can make the difference to this person between more misery or a way ahead. Listening, and therefore helping, is something active. It is a process, a journey. Any journey is easier when you know where you want to go and you have a plan of how to get there. Many people have set out various models for such a journey. They put different phases on different aspects of this journey. Thus all the models are similar, but not quite the same. They present different means of helping another person to take that journey more confidently and under his or her own steam. As such, the models have advantages and disadvantages, and comparing them can be useful so that you can see which one would be most appropriate for you when you help other people.

When there is a model or framework, and when both helper

Table 4.1. Different models for helping

Egan	Carkhuff	Nelson-Jones		Tschudin
1. Present scenario Story Blind spots	Attending Responding to clients Feelings Reason	D	Develop the relationship, identify and clarify problem(s)	What is happening?
		A	Access problem(s) and redefine in skills terms	
Leverage	Personalizing the experience Meaning			What is the meaning of it?
2. Preferred scenario Possibilities Agenda Commitment	Goal	S	State working goals and plan interventions	What is your goal?
3. Getting there Strategies Best fit Plan	Initiating action	I	Intervene to develop self-helping skills	How are you going to do it?
		E	End and consolidate self-helping skills	

and client know that model, then the work done will be more focused, more satisfying, and a goal will possibly be identified and reached more quickly. Models are useful to keep to the task in hand. And they are useful for training in counselling skills, and to refer to when 'stuck' or 'lost' during a conversation, in order to find a fresh perspective.

A model has to be simple to understand and simple to use. Nelson-Jones (1993, p. 30) found that his trainees could not easily remember his model, but when he produced the acronym DASIE (see Table 4.1) they could remember the stages.

Just as each patient and client is different, so each helper is different. Which theory and/or model you use is eventually less important than that you use it confidently, and your clients are helped effectively by it.

Different theories

This book is more concerned with the practical application of counselling skills than with the underlying theories of psychology and therapy. A basic knowledge of human nature, illness and approaches to therapy are taken for granted. Some of the theories of counselling are well known: Gestalt therapy (Perls, 1973), transactional analysis (TA) (Berne, 1964; Harris, 1973), client- or person-centred therapy (Rogers, 1951), rational emotive therapy (RET) (Ellis, 1962), behavioural therapy (Krumboltz and Thorenson, 1969), neuro-linguistic programming (NLP) (Bandler, 1985), reality therapy (Glasser, 1965) and psychosynthesis (Ferrucci, 1982). Readers who are interested in knowing more about these theories in the context of counselling are referred in particular to Nelson-Jones (1982) and Hough (1994), to the annotated bibliography in Chapter 15, and to libraries and bookshops for specific titles relating to the therapy in question.

Different models

Table 4.1 shows four different approaches to helping. They are laid out in such a way that the reader can easily see where they coincide. It may also be helpful to compare these with the nursing process:

1. Assessment
2. Planning
3. Implementation
4. Evaluation.

But there is one big difference between the models for helping and the nursing process: the models are all directed to problem *management*, but the nursing process is oriented towards problem *solving*. This should not be overlooked.

On the whole, nurses are people who are problem-solving oriented: they see a nursing problem, identify it, and set out to resolve it. But counselling is different. In helping and counselling, the focus is on the individual, not the problem. In helping we are dealing with a person: a person with a problem. For most nurses, this will represent a drastic change of emphasis.

The person presents a problem, but the problem is not the focus. If it is, then the process used is either advising or information giving. A problem has a *solution*; counselling works towards a *goal*. Counselling helps the *person*, and that normally means focusing on the person's *feelings* first of all, and then on the *meaning* of these feelings for the person.

The models outlined are therefore problem-management models because the person has to learn to manage a problem, not necessarily solve it. These aspects should become clearer as you read through the book, particularly when concentrating on the skills.

Counselling exists to *help*, that is, to help individuals focus on a goal or outcome. That still means that there is a process and something has to move. But the difference between counselling and the nursing process is that there is not necessarily a problem to be solved in counselling; rather there is a goal to work towards. The process in counselling is *similar* to the nursing process, but it is not identical.

Egan's model

Gerard Egan's model of helping (1994) has evolved and changed considerably over the twenty years in which his book has been widely used. Egan sees his model to be a problem-management/opportunity-development approach to helping; it is 'an open systems model', universal and also eclectic. He describes a three-stage model with each stage further divided into three steps. These steps combine for action, leading to valued outcomes.

Stage 1: Reviewing the current scenario. The principle here is to 'help clients identify, explore and clarify their problem situations and unused opportunities' (p. 22). Clients are clients because they are stuck in a particular situation from which they cannot extricate themselves and which they find painful or problematic.

Stage 2: Developing the preferred scenario. The principle behind this stage is that clients are helped to 'identify what they want in terms of goals and objectives that are based on an understanding of problem situations and opportunities' (p. 22). When clients have a better view of their problems they will be able to understand better what their options are. This stage looks at outcomes and possible results.

Stage 3: Getting there. The principle here is to help clients 'develop strategies for accomplishing goals, for getting what they want' (p. 22). The gap between knowing what one wants and getting it can, however, be rather large. 'Getting there' is helping the client to narrow the gap to something manageable.

These stages are then each divided into three steps. In Stage 1 clients are helped to tell their story; to identify any blind spots which prevent them from seeing the problem or opportunities; and to identify and work on problems or issues that will make a difference. Egan uses the term 'leverage' to mean gaining an advantage or having a handle with which to steer in the desired direction.

Stage 2 develops the preferred scenario by considering the possibilities for a better future; translating these possibilities into viable goals; and then being committed to a programme of constructive change. If this sounds very involved and complicated, it need not be. In order to outline what is happening in the process, there is always a good deal of theory involved which in actual life may be reduced to just a few words.

If Stage 2 deals with *what* clients want, Stage 3 deals with *how* they get there. The first principle here is to consider various strategies; choosing which strategy fits best; and finally turning strategies into a plan of action. In this way, the whole process leads to outcomes that are valued.

In an earlier model Egan (1986) had seen the process as a circle with 'evaluation' in the middle. The latest model consists of three semi-circles, rather like question marks facing the wrong way, but there is an 'E' in the centre of the semi-circles, indicating that evaluation takes place constantly. Unless there is adjustment to what is going on at every level, helping may be quite ineffective.

Egan is not at all dogmatic about his model. He does not say that because of this model clients actually end up managing both problems and opportunities better. It is up to the clients to live more effectively or not. He does not think that dragging clients mechanistically through the stages and steps of the model is helpful. At any given moment a client may be at any one or more stages and steps, and helpers need to be flexible enough to help creatively.

Carkhuff's model

Robert Carkhuff (1987) calls his theoretical approach a 'developmental model for helping'. His basic premise is that 'to live is to grow'. Depending on what we can do for ourselves, what others do for us, or what we do for others at crisis points in life is 'for better or for worse'. How we help at such crisis points is therefore crucial if it is to be for the better, i.e. for growing.

The three goals of helping, according to Carkhuff, are exploration, understanding and action. These combine in a process which recycles itself. Through action comes feedback, which leads to further exploration, and that in turn sets the stage for more accurate self-understanding. Into this setting come his four stages of helping: attending, responding, personalizing the experience and initiating action.

Attending is being with individual clients both physically and psychologically. We are with them verbally and non-verbally. The key ingredient of attending is listening.

Responding means hearing the client's words, but also being aware of behaviours and feelings. As these come to the fore, the helpers respond, i.e. point them out, feed them back to clients, make them obvious and give clients the possibility to see, hear and feel their own ways of being.

Personalizing the experience is making the step from 'it happened because of. . .' to 'it happened because I. . .'. When clients are able to take responsibility for actions and feelings, then they will be more able to change because arbitrary forces are no longer working on them: they themselves will make things happen. This can be understood clearly only when clients have seen the meaning and sense in these forces, and understand them in terms of themselves, i.e. personally.

Initiating action is the goal and also the first step along a new and different way of being. Carkhuff said that the goal is like the 'flip' side of the problem: when the problem is turned over, the goal is there! This is essentially what helping is about, and Carkhuff's model aims to do this by the above four steps.

Nelson-Jones' model

Richard Nelson-Jones (1993, p. 33) intends that helpers and clients should collaborate to attain the goals at each stage of his 'Lifeskills Helping Model'. This is done with helpers and clients using both 'thinking skills' and 'action skills' at every stage of the process.

Stage 1: **D**evelop the relationship, identify and clarify problem(s). The task is to 'build rapport and help clients to reveal, identify and describe problem(s)'.

Stage 2: **A**ssess problem(s) and redefine in skills terms. In this stage the task is to 'elicit relevant information to define problem(s) in skills terms'.

Stage 3: State working goals and plan interventions. Working goals should now be stated and self-helping interventions negotiated to attain them.

Stage 4: Intervene to develop self-helping skills. The task is now 'to work to develop self-helping skills strengths in problem areas'.

Stage 5: End and consolidate self-helping skills. The helping contact is terminated and self-helping skills are consolidated.

Nelson-Jones talks about 'lifeskills helping'. He says that 'lifeskills helping aims to articulate the "common sense" of effective helping'. This model is firmly people-centred. He prefers to think of people as possessing skills strengths or skills weaknesses rather than having skills or not having them. He has therefore drawn his philosophy together into a definition of lifeskills:

Lifeskills are personally responsible sequences of self-helping choices in specific psychological skills areas conducive to mental wellness. People require a repertoire of lifeskills according to their developmental tasks and specific problems of living. (Nelson-Jones, 1993, p. 30)

The Four Questions

Over many years of counselling practice, inside and outside nursing, I have developed my own model for helping and counselling in the form of four questions. This will be outlined in detail in Chapter 5. The Four Questions are:

What is happening?
What is the meaning of it?
What is your goal?
How are you going to do it?

The stages of counselling

So that the models may be seen to have practical application, I shall describe here the stages, as outlined in Table 4.1, related to a specific example.

In a chapter entitled 'The myth and reality of interpersonal skills use in nursing', Cormack (1985) gives an example of interactions between a patient and his nurses. It is an anecdote of 'a young man who had to be hospitalized for medical treatment of an eye ailment'.

I shall first quote the story and then, with the help of the models, imagine what the specific counselling interactions might have been like.

The impatience of the man during this, his first, hospitalization, coupled with a natural shyness and feeling of inferiority, resulted in considerable anxiety and reluctance to stay for the duration of his treatment. When asked why he did stay and complete the treatment, he replied: 'It was because of the nurses. They made me feel welcome, they made me feel at home. After a while, they made me feel just like one of them. They made me want to stay and finish the treatment.'

The story says that the patient was shy, feeling inferior, anxious and reluctant to be in hospital.

First of all, in *attending* (Carkhuff) to patients or clients you show that you are aware of body language, feelings that are around, facts you know, and anything else that presents itself. You notice these, but you do not judge the person with you because of them. You are, and stay, with the person. You don't just say 'Good morning' as you pass the foot of their bed, but you go up to them. You give them your time, your attention, your energy, your knowledge. For the time being this person alone matters. When this person has your attention then he or she also concentrates on what is going on.

I imagine a conversation between this patient and a nurse could have started something like:

Patient: I don't think this treatment is helping me.
Nurse: What makes you think so?
Patient: It's done nothing for me so far and I feel a fraud taking up a bed.
Nurse: I don't consider you to be a fraud, but do I suspect a bit of impatience?
Patient: A bit of it? A great deal of it!
Nurse: Do you think your eyes are worth waiting for a day or two to see how the treatment goes?
Patient: All right, you win. Put like this, sure, they are worth waiting for.

This interaction simply shows that, by giving attention to the person, much can be achieved. If the nurse had simply replied 'Patience, man, patience!' to the original statement, he might have felt patronized and been even more ready to leave, but the attention he got showed him that the nurse cared for him as a person, and that made him want to stay.

In terms of the models, this interaction represented:

Present scenario: story, blind spots (Egan)
Develop the relationship, identify and clarify the problem(s)
   (Nelson-Jones)
Responding to clients (feelings, reason) (Carkhuff)
What is happening? (Tschudin)

In any situation in which you need to get somewhere, it is best to know where you are starting from. In counselling, this means that clients have to describe the problem. This is often not easy at all.

I don't know what's happening to me.
I seem to have lost my grip of things.
It's like being in a tunnel without any light at the end.

These and similar statements seem to be more common than

I know exactly what I need (or want).

Very often, people find an 'obvious' problem as an entry to asking for help. This can be conscious and deliberate, wanting to see how helpers will respond before they expose their heart. It can also be a subconscious ploy so as *not* to look deeper.

I've got such a headache today.
If only this swallowing would improve, then I'd be perfectly all right.

Imagine that the example patient might have said:

I've never been in hospital before; I don't know how to fit into a routine.

These are all opening gambits and they may be the problem which patients want to come to terms with. This may well not be the 'real' problem. For clients to voice their real problems, and for helpers to hear them, a story needs to be told. This is often therapeutic in itself. A person may have been thinking over a problem, turning it round and round in the mind and never coming to a real conclusion. In *telling* it to someone who hears and responds, a solution can present itself.

Sometimes there seem to be layers and layers of problems. One problem identified leads to half a dozen more to be discovered. At this stage the important element is to voice the problems, become aware of them and describe them.

Egan calls this 'the present scenario': that which is happening now. In this stage the story is told, and the helper, trying to hear what is happening, listens for significant words or phrases, and for what seem to be blind spots. The important thing at this stage is to hold the problem in the present, and to work on it.

As well as setting a working frame for the counselling process, Carkhuff has also established four essential features within that model:

1. Feeling
2. Reason
3. Meaning
4. Goal.

This makes it clear that, if you want to help a person, then what matters most are the *feelings*. Most people have difficulties with their feelings. They live entirely from their feelings and cannot be rational, or they deny their feelings and 'think' their way out of a problem. When we learn how to deal with feelings, then problems can usually be dealt with because they are no longer a threat. But this is easier said than done.

Identifying the main or important feeling in a story is not always easy. Because the person tells a story, it will usually be the *facts* that are concentrated on. Facts give the tangible points of reference within which life happens. To respond appropriately to the person at this stage is therefore always to search for the feelings. This, simply put, is what responding empathically is about.

Feelings are never isolated. There is always a reason. And that reason constitutes the story. What happened for this feeling to exist? What is happening now to the client as she or he is telling the story? What feelings does the story-telling engender?

A different interaction between the example patient and nurse might have been, starting with the same opening statement:

Patient: I don't think this treatment is helping me.
Nurse: What makes you think so?
Patient: It's done nothing for me so far and I feel a fraud taking up a bed.
Nurse: A fraud?

Patient: Well, yes, there's nothing really wrong with me that should keep me in hospital.

Nurse: It sounds as if you would rather not be here.

Patient: I can hardly stand it. Seeing all these other people around me gives me the shivers.

Nurse: You've never seen so many ill people before all together?

Patient: No, and I think it's going to be me next going blind.

Nurse: You sound as if you are really afraid of being blind.

Patient: I had never voiced it before, but yes, I know, that's what it's all about.

Nurse: Do you want to tell me about it?

Patient: I have always been too scared to face it but I can't avoid it now. Yes, do you have the time?

A real counselling conversation would probably have more interaction, but this shows the general direction of helping and counselling in this, the opening stage.

In this example the nurse picked up (showing empathy) that the patient was afraid of going blind. The feeling is fear, and by voicing this she was right into the main problem. She had responded correctly, and the patient was then ready to tell her his story. He could begin to give the reason for his feelings.

In the terms of the models, this interaction showed:

Access the problem(s) (Nelson-Jones).
Personalizing the experience (Carkhuff).
Leverage (Egan).
What is the meaning of it? (Tschudin).

One of the most useful things that helpers can do is to enable clients to see their problem in the context of life. A problem never appears out of the blue and, however much it may seem to be unrelated to other spheres of life, a few simple connections will usually give a totally different picture. Once this happens there is a sense of 'aha!' and some form of meaning can be attached to the problem.

Once a problem has been named, it needs to be accepted as one's own. It needs to be made personal; scapegoats are no longer valid. The notion of self-responsibility has to come into the picture.

They give me the shivers.
You make me so angry.
She shouldn't be allowed to do this to people.

These and similar statements are usually around at the beginning of a helping interaction. Clients are behaving as victims. In order now to tackle the problem, clients have to learn that the only people who are victims are those who allow themselves to be victims. Nobody *makes* them angry, but *they are* angry.

Nelson-Jones refers to skills deficits which have to be seen and identified; Egan calls them blind spots. The original problem can now be related to other areas of behaviour or attitudes. Patterns can be seen which put the problem into a wider context. Has this happened before? What did you do then?

This leads to the meaning. Is this problem a defence mechanism? Does it protect something? Does it stop the person from functioning well now? Is it something that should be let go, forgiven or 'unlearned'? Is it something that has been hidden for a long time but now cannot be hidden any longer? What is the name for the problem?

It is often a necessary step at this stage to help patients or clients to get deeply in touch with the morass in which they find themselves. This morass is usually so uncomfortable that clients would give anything to be rid of it. Nevertheless, without having owned it, recognized responsibility for it, and thus chosen to move forward, there is never going to be a clear goal. It is a measure of the helper's skills to stay with clients in this uncomfortable place and support them through it. Most people know instinctively that when they come to a wall, climbing over it, skirting round it or digging under it are not real solutions; but finding a door or gate is. The morass will end when such an opening has been located.

The 'problem' has now become only an identity-tag for the work that the person is doing. Because the person recognizes that what matters are the presenting feelings and how they hinder or help, she or he is no longer afraid and paralysed, but able to function more fully. Nelson-Jones calls this redefining the problem in skills terms.

Imagine what the example patient might now be telling the nurse:

Patient: Do you have time to listen?

Nurse: I am all ears.

Patient: Well, where to begin? There was this boy at school ... My grandmother was almost blind for years ... She couldn't really cope, but she refused help ... She impressed me both by her independence and by the way her clothes were always stained with food.

Nurse: Having an eye problem now makes you relate to her and you

	think one day you will be stubborn and off-putting to others by wearing food-stained clothes?
Patient:	You guessed!
Nurse:	Have you ever been in such a situation?
Patient:	Well, you could say I am now; I don't fit in here, and I wanted to go home, and I can't see enough with this treatment, so I may spill tea or toothpaste down my front.
Nurse:	I sense that you are afraid of losing control, and also of having to conform.
Patient:	I am afraid of getting old, of being ill, and not having achieved anything in my life.

The new 'problem' that emerges here is the fear of blindness. This is what Egan means by 'leverage': finding what is behind the obvious gives the problem a 'handle'. Carkhuff calls this 'personalizing the experience'. Whereas the initial problem was that the patient did not want to stay in hospital, it becomes evident that he might have wanted to escape having to face his feelings of fear and loss of control. This is the meaning of the problem: once the patient can see that this is the core of his shyness, feelings of inferiority, anxiety and reluctance to stay, he will see himself and his world in a different light.

Having come to some insight, there has to be some movement to 'ground' or actualize this experience. The interaction would probably have gone on for a while but, sooner or later, the counsellor has to point out that the client has to do something with his insight: what is his goal now? Where does he go from here?

The various models call this:

Preferred scenario: possibilities (Egan).
Initiating action (Carkhuff).
State working goals (Nelson-Jones).
What is your goal? (Tschudin).

Having become aware of the problem and internalized it by paying attention to it, the next step is one of choice.

Egan (1994, p. 220) says that at this stage the question is: 'What do you want?' This is a question which is not often asked by helpers. My guess is that the question is not often asked because the assumption is that the helper has to give something that is impossible, and the client expects to be given something – preferably something life-changing. Therefore it is better to avoid such a question. Egan makes it clear that this first question has to be followed by a second, equally direct, question: 'What do you have to do to get what you want?'

The *preferred scenario* here is to consider possibilities, look for an agenda and ask the client for a commitment to this scenario.

In an earlier edition (1986), Egan places emphasis on imagination at this stage. It is therefore interesting to note that he has moved to a more direct approach with clients. This is similar to the Four Questions model which will be outlined in more detail in later chapters. Imagination is still necessary and valid, but a direct question is more searching and clients are less able to divert attention and avoid dealing with what they have already partly tackled. Since avoidance (or entropy, as Egan calls it; see Chapter 9) is common at this stage, direct questions are another reason to be helpful.

Carkhuff, who puts his emphasis on development and growing, also sees developing goals as the aim of the helping process.

Nelson-Jones writes of choosing and negotiating interventions. He believes that goals should involve individuals, singly or collectively, and be guided by our values and understanding of human nature (Nelson-Jones, 1982, p. 190). Therefore our goals are conditioned as well as free, conscious as well as unconscious. They may be practical goals, but they are also psychological. As always, an integration of all aspects will lead to a more holistic outcome.

The counsellor's skills have been important all the time, but at this stage they become particularly evident. It is all too easy to slip into the advising mode:

If I were you I would. . .
What you need to do is. . .

This simply highlights the helper's goals, not those of the client. This is something that must be kept firmly in mind, as otherwise the process can no longer be said to be 'helping', but becomes advice. Carkhuff is adamant that helping is always 'for better or for worse' but is never neutral. It is for better or for worse here mainly because of the helper's skills.

The essence of this stage is therefore 'the preferred scenario'. Possibilities are considered. It is important here to challenge the 'one-track mind'. The fact that perhaps only one solution was ever considered before might have created the whole problem. To think creatively now can help 'unmake' the problem. To help clients to achieve this, strategies like brainstorming and using force-field analysis may be helpful. Helpers may also use examples of how other people have tackled such problems, and indeed use self-disclosure, that is, 'how it worked for me'. This must be done sensitively though, because it could be seen as 'because it worked for me it will also work for you' and clients may think or feel that it should work for them because the counsellors are in a position of authority or reverence. These aspects will be dealt with in later chapters. The basis of the helper's interventions should always be support, and a firm belief in the client's ability to cope and manage.

Look at the example patient again, and imagine in your own mind how this goal-setting might be achieved. In my own words, they may be saying something like this to each other, picking the conversation up where it left before:

Patient: I am afraid of getting old, of being ill, and not having achieved anything in my life.

Nurse: There is another fear now, that of getting old. And there is a fear of not using your life fully.

Patient: The fear of getting old and being ill is quite overpowering.

Nurse: Do you equate being old and being ill?

Patient: To an extent, yes.

Nurse: You are ill now, but you are not old.

Patient: I hadn't thought of it that way. Perhaps that's why I am impatient now, because I am not old, but I feel old and helpless with this illness.

Nurse: You are touching on more and more aspects of yourself. Which do you think is the one that matters most at this moment?

Patient: Well – right now, I think, being impatient.

Nurse: What are you therefore looking for at this moment?

Patient: To have patience and cope with this treatment.

Nurse: It sounds quite easy. Is it?

Patient: Yes and no. You are helping me to see that it could be less difficult than I thought.

Nurse: Can you see a way of putting 'being patient' into practice?

Patient: Saying it like this makes it possible to tackle it. Being more patient – yes, that's what it is. That might also put the other issues and fears into a more manageable perspective.

Again, this is not how a 'real' conversation would go. There would probably be many more interactions in between. Perhaps also some pauses, questions, 'don't know's and encouraging 'um's and a good deal of body language which can be revealing of a person's feelings. However, the general trend can be seen. The patient is gradually working towards owning the feelings, taking responsibility for them, moving forward by seeing some meaning for his feelings and present uncomfortable state, and finally doing something to get out of the morass on to more comfortable and sure ground.

Having had to go over the same or similar ground more than once by looking at the various feelings that presented themselves, and having had goals in sight, this example of the conversation is now getting to the stage of a clear goal emerging. In the words of the models:

Getting there (Egan).
Initiating action (Carkhuff).
Intervene to develop self-helping skills (Nelson-Jones).
How are you going to do it? (Tschudin).

Yet even the best-laid plan may come to nothing if it is not carried out. This may be simple enough when it is a question of putting on a party or building a house, but when it means changing an attitude or acting differently towards a person, it may be much more difficult. It will, after all, mean a turning around of a part of one's life. Therefore it is vitally important that this stage is included in any model of helping.

However well goals are set and perhaps tried out, most people meet some difficulty. The clients who have learnt to be more assertive and now set forth to *be* assertive will still find occasionally that it is difficult, and make a mistake. That is the moment when clients need support and perhaps more help in re-examining the goals and re-negotiating interventions. Therefore, to spell out again how the goal is put into practice is always a good and helpful point.

Patient: Being more patient – yes, that's what it is.
Nurse: That's a very good point. How are you going to do it?
Patient: By telling myself to be patient.
Nurse: It sounds as if this is just a bit too easy – as if you always tell yourself to be patient.
Patient: (astonished) You are reading me like a book! Yes, I often tell myself to be patient, and, come to think of it, I usually end up being more impatient than before.
Nurse: So how are you going to be patient now?
Patient: I am going to stay here and I'm going to see the treatment through. And I'm not going to moan but I'm going to be positive about it because you helped me see the point of it all. Can I help *you* with anything around the ward?

A good helping relationship has a good beginning, middle and end. Each aspect is important. Sadly, the end is often a neglected area. Good endings make for good memories, and these nourish us in times of doubt and less success. Nurses feel very satisfied when a dressing is well done or a patient is made comfortable in a difficult position. When the position is one of the heart and the mind, the end is no less important.

The interaction that I have traced through this chapter is a one-off, short episode. There will be many of these in every nurse's work; but there will also be long-term relationships.

The example I used concentrated first on fear, and then became more immediate by focusing on impatience. Fear is something so common that it underlies many of our behaviours and attitudes. But the other, and just as strong, element in most people's lives is loss. Being ill is then another loss. Being helped by counselling is a restoration, but having that help terminated or withdrawn may bring the whole problem back again and even make it worse. The ending of a relationship is therefore crucial, and may need to be carefully prepared.

Imagine the example patient one more time:

Patient: I'm going to stay here... Can I help you with anything around the ward?

Nurse: By staying you are actually helping yourself and me too – we are only two sides of one coin! By helping me – that's great, you show that you are serious about what we just discussed. Can you sit with P. for a while. He feels a bit lonely.

Patient: You mean doing to him what you just did to me?

Nurse: Sort of, yes!

Patient: I'm not a counsellor.

Nurse: You don't have to be, but he said something about the day being long this morning.

Patient: I get the point: patience!

Nurse: It was your idea... I'm around if you need help.

This extract shows a form of ending, and also how self-help skills can be consolidated. The aim of counselling is that the client can live more resourcefully and satisfyingly or, in other words, get along without a helper. The nurse encouraged this patient to do so straight away, and practising is the best way to prove that what you preach is valid.

Making this, the last stage in the helping relationship, right is important for the client as well as for the helper. A relationship left open, unfinished and perhaps painful, is always difficult. It is not always possible to leave your clients on a 'high', but to leave them floundering may be destructive. Leaving clients quietly crying may be all right in some circumstances; leaving them in a rage may not. But simply plastering over cracks may not be all right either. A relationship is really ended only when the feelings of both parties are OK, and for that to happen you have to be responsible for your own feelings.

Models for counselling are useful in that they give guidelines and boundaries. But these guidelines and boundaries have to be flexible and imaginative. In the example conversations there was no use of jargon or of any of the words with which the various stages are described. A helpful interaction is not a set piece. What matters most of all is that one human being has been helped by another, and both are benefiting from this helping – one by being helped, the other by giving effectively.

CHAPTER FIVE

The Four Questions

....

The background to the Four Questions model

I have always used a model to help me keep to a direction in counselling. Without some signposts I find that I – like many others – can get waylaid by the problem instead of concentrating on the person. This can result in ineffective helping. The clients and I both realize that and both feel frustrated.

If a model is too long, or too complicated, it is not much use to me, because the model detracts from the person. When I discovered the simple four-word model of Carkhuff, I felt I could use it, but still be free to be myself. I did not have to think of stages any more. Yet I felt concerned that there was nothing in that model about putting insights into practice. Simply having a 'goal' is like a New Year's resolution: it is not based on anything concrete, spelled out and with a personal commitment. The main aim of counselling is to help a person to change in some way, and the leap between insight and practical change being carried out is perhaps the most difficult thing to do, and why so many of us are happier to stay with 'the devil we know'. If counselling is successful then we can not only name 'the devil' that plagues us, but see it for what it is and deal with it in an appropriate way and then experience the freedom which this brings.

The four questions evolved and emerged from other people's writings, from what I heard myself say to clients, from management strategies I met, and perhaps even from my unconscious, because one morning they seemed just to be there, perfectly obvious.

1. What is happening?
2. What is the meaning of it?
3. What is your goal?
4. How are you going to do it?

The reasons for questions

Some of the advantages of having a model in the form of questions are:

a) The questions are simple and easily remembered.

b) Asking the client these specific questions helps you, the helper, to concentrate on the client, not on your own need to keep to a model.

c) Questions keep the focus on the client.

d) Questions make clients work. You are less likely to propose your own solutions, but help clients to find their own goals.

e) These questions are not exclusive; many other questions can and need to be asked as well.

f) The questions do not have to be used in the form given here. Helpers can and should find their own ways of expressing them in different circumstances and situations.

g) The questions can be models for other questions in the process.

h) These questions can also be used for your own evaluation of a session, or process, and can be helpful for supervision.

What is happening?

What is happening is the first question at the beginning of a relationship. The person who says:

I am not feeling well.
I have had quite a week.
I've got some good news.
Guess what's happened to me.
Things are not going well.

wants to tell a story, and the helper invites the story to be told.

In such circumstances it is clear that the actual question 'What is happening?' is not necessarily asked at all. Our skills of communicating with each other are perfectly adequate to say something like: 'well. . .', 'tell me then. . .', or some remark that invites the speaker to elaborate. The question 'What is happening?' is in this instance merely a reminder that this is the opening or beginning of a helping situation or relationship. The starting point is the present, and this needs to be captured. 'What is happening?' therefore points to the need to concentrate on the present.

The question 'What is happening?' here marks the first stage of helping. Since this is usually a long stage compared with the others, there are various aspects to this question.

The helper invites the person to talk   Sometimes a person is bursting to tell a story, at other times there is reluctance. If the question 'What is happening?' is asked directly, the helper invites the client to say more.

The question shows a non-judgemental attitude Simply asking such an open question shows that the listener is ready to hear whatever may be said. This implies a prior willingness to listen and an attitude of being willing to share time with this person.

The client is sure to be listened to When a clear signal has been given to a client to talk, that client is assured of being heard. This is affirmation of the client as a person.

The helper needs information To help realistically, the helper needs a good deal of information, which must be given. To make sense of another person's life, we relate ourselves to events, and these have to be detailed. The helper needs to hear these details to respond helpfully.

A wider picture has to emerge It is not only factual details that the helper has to understand, but a complex picture of a person has to emerge. In this way, 'What is happening?' takes on a wider meaning.

What is going on here?
What is the person saying or not saying?
What is the story about?
How is the story being told?
What body language is displayed?
What feelings are expressed?
What does the client reveal?
What might the client conceal?
What blind spots might there be?
What energy is evident?

These are aspects of the first question which may go through the helper's mind as the client talks, and to each aspect the question 'What is happening?' may be applied, either spoken or unspoken.

The helper's own questioning As the helper listens, there are aspects of the story that are picked up and noticed, but which the helper may not ask in so many words:

What am I really hearing?
What am I not hearing?

What vibes are around?
What is happening to me as I listen to this story?
What reactions do I have as I listen?
What is going on between the client and myself?
What feelings do I have for this client?
What sort of a relationship is there between us?
What might I be conveying to the client?

The question 'What is happening?' can be very useful for
the sort of internal checking that goes on as we talk. Thus the
question can be asked *to* the client and *about* the client, and
also *to* ourselves and *about* the relationship.

In the course of a helping situation, short or long, this question may have to be asked many times. As new facets come
to life, they have to be explained and explored, and 'What is
happening?' gives each of them time and space in which to
develop. The fact that this is an open question makes the process one of helping rather than advising. All the aspects of
helping are also constantly reviewed in this way.

The question takes on different aspects if the different
words are emphasized differently:

What is happening?
What *is* happening?
What is *happening*?

Perhaps the greatest obstacle to helping and good relationships in general is the making of assumptions. We assume that
the other person knows what we know or thinks as we think.
One way in which this can be overcome is by asking open
questions. When it concerns helping, then open questions –
at least to begin with – are essential. 'What is happening?' is
such a question.

What is the meaning of it?

When there has been some discussion and evaluation of the
situation presented by the client, there comes a point at which
some insight has to be gained before the client can move on.
After all, a problem exists because the client is stuck in some
way, cannot see beyond a certain point, or perhaps fear and
anger prevent a way forward.

This question is more particularly relevant in actual counselling situations than in circumstances when only the skills of
counselling are used. If there is only a short interaction and
all that is required is a new view of a problem, the question
does not necessarily apply. The person who has a headache

because of some worry which causes tension may not at that moment need or be willing to examine the wider and deeper implications of that tension. A person who is willing to hear the story behind the headache may give the client enough space to cope with the headache and the situation adequately – at least this time. It is inappropriate to probe into the client's psyche to find some deep-seated problem if this is not wanted or needed. It is even more inappropriate to do this simply to satisfy a model. In this situation counselling skills will have been used, but counselling as such will not have taken place.

In most helping situations, though, there is a need to 'anchor' an insight gained when the first question has been asked and answered adequately. Egan (1994, p. 27) speaks of 'leverage' at this stage, and Carkhuff (1987, p. 14) points out that 'personalizing the experience' is now called for. A kind of 'internalizing' has to take place before a new image or vision can emerge and change can happen. This is perhaps best illustrated by the client no longer saying 'it (or he or she) makes me so angry' but realizing that 'I am angry'. An internal adaptation has taken place and thus a meaning has been acknowledged. It is no longer some other force that moves a person, but the source of the force is seen to be inside.

This question needs to be understood in a very wide sense. A young man who has been badly hurt in a motorcycle accident may have difficulty in seeing any meaning in the accident. If, however, he is gradually able to live with any disability, then he may begin to see that his life can have a different meaning from the one he might have imagined before the accident. A 50-year-old woman with breast cancer, on the other hand, may find that having cancer has given new meaning to her personally in that she sees the cancer as the trigger to self-awareness, self-knowledge and self-assertiveness. For her, cancer has meaning.

'What is the meaning of it?' should be taken as that moment when a client comes to understanding or insight:

'Ah, I see. . .'
'Yes, that makes sense. . .'
'The point of this is. . .'

This question basically looks for a connection between the obvious and the hidden, and between what is and what might be. It may therefore have to be asked in many different ways:

What significance does the problem have in your life?
What memories does this bring up?

What patterns do you detect?
What purpose is there in the problem?
What purpose is there in seeking help?
What sense do you see here?
How do you interpret what is going on?
What insights have you come to?
Is there a light somewhere? What is it?

'What is the meaning of it?' tries to elicit purpose and sense in order to understand. If we know the 'why' of a problem, we can usually tolerate a great deal of 'how', that is, we can put up with pain and discomfort if we know that it is going to be of use in the long run.

For most people, illness and suffering present a moment of truth, and this question will help them to make sense of this 'moment'. Finding a meaning in life, suffering and death is a crucial element not just for patients and clients, but for any of us who are around sick people, especially if we try to help them. The meaning changes from time to time, particularly when some disaster has happened. It is then that life and living have to be reinterpreted, and asking this question may then be the crucial one.

Finding meaning is not always what clients want or search for. We cannot give them meaning, and we cannot make them want to have or find meaning. Just as some people will not come to an acceptance of loss or disability, so some people do not want to gain insights. This has to be respected and not judged as wrong. Nevertheless, the question does need to be asked, in some form or another, in order to help realistically.

This stage is approached again with a question; this is deliberate. As we work with people and listen to their stories, it is very easy to think, 'He just has to be more tolerant'; 'She must be firm'; 'If only he were not so lazy'; 'Why on earth did she do this?' In other words, we imagine or assume that we have the solution to their problems. Many of us are not backwards in coming forward with them. Nelson-Jones (1993, p. 5) distinguishes between private and public talk in counselling. The above statements are examples of the private 'self-talk' of helpers. The public talk is inevitably coloured by the private talk. The public talk consists of 'action skills'; the skills of counselling. The private talk is what might be equated with the attitudes or core conditions of helpers. The private talk is therefore indicative of the warmth, genuineness and empathy of the helper. Thus, rather than making inappropriate self-talk public, asking a question may show that the actual attitude, that is, the question, is genuine and the self-talk is positive. Asking questions may also teach the helper to be genuinely warm and empathic.

In any kind of helping it is important to call forth what is there in the person rather than assume that there is nothing there. Helping is respecting the person, and, by asking, we respect their integrity.

As before, the question can be asked with different emphases:

What is the meaning of it?
What *is* the meaning of it?
What is the *meaning* of it?
What is the meaning of *it*?

Once an answer to the question of meaning has been given, a significant point has been reached. For any change to be possible, there has first to be an awareness, then an acknowledgement, and only then can change take place. When the client comes to acknowledgement, a meaning is often apparent. It has to be grasped and held, voiced, and in a way 'celebrated' because it is crucial. But just as one swallow does not make a summer, so an insight does not yet make change possible. The main aim of helping and counselling begins only now; the insight and understanding has to be transformed into some form of action or change.

What is your goal?

It would be so easy at this stage to say to the client, 'All you have to do is. . .'; or 'If you don't do. . .'; or worse still, 'If I were you, I would. . .'. We have all done this, and then seen the opposite being done, or nothing being done. It would then also be easy to say, 'I told you so' if the original problem persisted or got worse. But this means that we have not been effective helpers to begin with and therefore the other person has not been helped. The one thing that helping is not, is telling others what to do. We have no right to rule someone else's life, nor are others to live by our standards. Helping is about fostering in others their own resources to live more satisfyingly. Therefore, yet again, we ask a question: 'What is your goal now?'

For an insight to be meaningful, for an inspiration to be fruitful or for an intuition to be taken seriously, some change has to be made. The person who was looking for help wanted something to be different at the end of a talk or session. Clearly, some people think that the helper will do the changing for them. Part of the reason for asking for meaning is precisely so that clients realize they have to make the changes themselves. One of the phrases I most often say to clients is, 'You cannot change others; you can only change yourself'. In the same way, we as counsellors cannot change our clients. If they do not respond to our helping, we need to change our ways of helping them. (This is said with the proviso that there will always be some people who cannot be helped despite every effort made.)

What change is made clearly depends on the problem. Sometimes there is a simple answer to a complex problem. Many patients worry a great deal over some points of their illness or disease which can easily be explained by a nurse or doctor with some understanding of anatomy or physiology. Many changes that depend on a particular behaviour are fairly easy to make. Some training may be needed to change a behaviour, but, once learnt, there is a clear gain.

It is much more difficult to change attitudes: our own attitudes. Most of life's problems exist because of outmoded, irrelevant or blinkered attitudes held by us and others. We tend to see ourselves as victims of all kinds of powers which can rule our lives. When this has been acknowledged, we come to see ourselves not as victims any longer, nor necessarily as victors, but as partners with the flow of life, capable of changing the things we can change, leaving the things we cannot change – and knowing the difference between the two.

The goals that a client may work towards may be very different from what was presented as the main problem. This is mainly due to the fact that, if a meaning becomes evident, then it also becomes clear that an attitude is often the cause, and a goal may be to change that attitude. This shows the importance of the fact that it is a *goal* that is meant here, not a solution. A solution is something fixed and final. A goal is something to be achieved, and a possibility towards which clients can work. A person with multiple sclerosis cannot aim for elimination of the disease, but his or her goal may be to live more realistically with the disease when before he or she had been railing against the fate which allowed it to develop.

It is always the client's goal, never the helper's. This is perhaps one of the areas where it is important to have the empathy to understand what it might be like to be in a client's shoes, rather than trying to walk in their shoes ourselves. It is *so* easy to know what clients need to do, to offer a solution, and to tell them how to set about tidying up their life. But such things are our own aims and goals. This is a very strong reason why the question is addressed to the client and the client has to answer, not the helper. The skill of a helper is to tease out of a person what may be recognized as a goal.

Clients may hesitate to state a goal because it commits them, or because they believe that they may fail. Perhaps they are not used to thinking in terms of goals. Perhaps they think that goals are unrealistic. Particularly if someone is very ill, a goal may look like a fancy idea. Goals come in every shape and form. What matters is that the goal is realistic, however large or small, immediate or long-term.

Goals tend to present themselves in the course of conversation. It may be necessary for the helper to point out that something said may actually be a goal, or that something may be turned into a goal. Because the helper is not in the same situation as the client, he or she is able to have a slightly distanced view and may therefore be able to make suggestions. These suggestions may not necessarily be taken up, but they can help in forming the goal.

As with the other questions, the emphasis can be placed on any word in the question, and this may make a difference to how clients understand what is being asked:

What is your goal?
What *is* your goal?
What is *your* goal?
What is your *goal*?

The question may also be asked in many different ways:

Do you see any way forward from here?
What is your intention now?
Where does this leave you?
Is this a decision?
Do you have any aims for this?
How might this dream come true?
What potential do you see for your meaning?
Is there a purpose here?
What can you make of this?

The question 'What is your goal?' also delineates a stage of helping and is therefore a pointer to the stage as well as an actual question that can be asked.

Just as important as asking the question is the fact that the question may not need to be asked at all. If the helping so far has been good, or even adequate, then a goal may present itself quite logically. The helper is then nothing more (and nothing less) than the 'midwife' in the process.

Finding a goal is important in helping because it focuses the process and clients feel that the conversation has helped and been purposeful. Such conversations can be demanding and even painful. When clients realize that the demands made are for their own sake – not for the helper's – then it is easier to go along with the process.

A point of importance to realize is that goals are aims to achieve, but that sometimes they may never be achieved: they may never need to be achieved as they may change before this can happen. This is part of life's rich pattern of constant change. Often the journey matters much more than arriving at a destination. In that way the journey itself is the goal. There are plenty of people who are not on a journey: they are stuck at the moment. There are people who are on a backward journey, ruled by memories that cannot be changed. There are also people who are on a future journey, living in and for a future which is as yet unborn. Such people may find that stopping to examine life today – the moment of truth – is very daunting.

The goals that people recognize and pursue may be emotional, attitudinal or spiritual. But they are not just in the mind; they have to be translated into action of some kind.

How are you going to do it?

The question 'What is your goal?' anchors the meaning, and 'How are you going to do it?' will now anchor the goal.

This stage in the helping process is characterized by possibilities, strategies and plans. Using such words does not mean that the stage is full of management jargon. On the contrary, it is full of down-to-earth nitty-gritty practicalities. It may mean that a client has to speak to someone (perhaps even a husband or wife) about a subject that may be painful; it may be trying to see the world from a different perspective; it may be letting oneself go and enjoying a party; or not go to the party and stay at home deliberately. The possibilities are endless. Perhaps clients know exactly what is called for now. Or perhaps the helper has to provide some examples of what might be possible.

If a helper suggests to a client what may now be possible to carry out the goal, it must be clear that these are suggestions. The goal has to be appropriate, and neither too small to be discarded nor too big to be applied. It is unrealistic to think 'from tomorrow I will love Jane and all will be well' when there has been a relationship problem for years. Tomorrow may come and Jane may say just the wrong thing and the client will say to himself, 'Why was I such a fool as to believe that anything would be different?' and thus be disillusioned and disappointed. It may be more realistic to set as a goal: 'I would like to have a better relationship with Jane and for three days I am going to say one nice thing to her each day'. After three days this may be prolonged for another three days, or increased to two nice things per day.

The gap between the insight and the carrying out may be the longest journey for a person. It takes courage to be true to oneself, especially if this means changing an attitude. One of the reasons why helping and counselling is important for many people is that by stating a goal there is already a commitment made. What is said between two people creates a bond between them. The relationship the two people have becomes the basis for trust in oneself and in other people. Thus the relationship then also becomes the support that may be necessary to take the plunge to change. It will have been the ground in which meaning could be identified and goals nurtured and grown; now it sustains the action.

If helping has gone on between two people, the action is now entirely down to the client. All the plans and strategies should have encouraged and prepared the client to be able to act alone. It is clear that at this stage skills of self-helping will have had to be encouraged and fostered. The question 'How are you going to do it?' looks outwards and forwards. It is the question that prepares the ending of the relationship – or at least the ending of the relationship as it has existed so far.

One person may have several goals at once, or in sequence. This is possible, as long as the client knows which have priority or how they will be achieved together.

Sometimes it is necessary to ask any of the questions in the model several times until they are heard or addressed. So it may be that this question, too, has to be asked differently and more than once until it is clear that the client has answered it. At the same time it needs also to be said that the question need never be asked at all if the client states clearly what he or she is going to do without any prompting. But if the question has to be asked, it may be phrased in different ways:

What are you going to do about this?
How can you put this into practice?
How can you apply this in a practical way?
What are your priorities now?
What is your plan of action?
How will you monitor the outcome?

If there is a need to spell out the 'how?', it may be necessary to write this down, complete with date, time and actual action to be taken. This can be as elaborate or simple as desired. People who have difficulties with boundaries may need more detailed plans than those whose problems lie elsewhere.

The normal course of events would mean here that client and helper meet again after a crucial action has happened to evaluate the outcome. In practice this often may not happen. Where it is possible, though, it is also important that the helper does check with clients what happened, and that clients report accurately. This is mainly for purposes of support. The helper trusts clients to carry out what was agreed, and clients trust themselves to carry it out, but with the best will in the world the unforeseen cannot be catered for. If so, a new phase of helping starts.

There may be times when a helper knows simply from the way a client said something that this person will change in the way outlined. It may then not be necessary to add details of how, where and when. The trust between the two people is enough. Or perhaps the insight was strong enough to provide the impulse for the change. The skills of clients and helpers differ, but both need to rely on the skills they have and trust their judgement.

A model for helping is useful. When you know the basics, however, they become part of you and you have no need to refer back to the model or theory. The point of helping is that clients become more resourceful and satisfied with living. In the same way, when models have taught you all there is to know about them, as a helper you can be more resourceful and your practice becomes more satisfactory for you. Use this or any other model, therefore, as long as it helps, but discard it once you feel competent enough – and perhaps able enough – to use your own model.

CHAPTER SIX

The components of helping

....

The setting

The counselling and helping done by nurses is unique in that it takes place within the context of physical and mental illness and pain, but, as every nurse knows, this is only the most obvious and practical part of helping. What cannot be so easily seen and touched is just as real: the suffering within the person who is ill. With more and more emphasis on holistic care and primary nursing, it is clear that both these aspects need to be taken into account. Salvage (1990) cites research which found that 'patients judged the quality of nursing by its emotional style', that is, by the nurses' awareness of patients' practical and *emotional* needs, and their response to both.

Some patients may be very ill and unable to be even partially self-caring, being passive recipients of care without the ability to express any emotions, but still aware of themselves as persons, not just bodies to be serviced.

Other patients may simply be passing through. With more and more emphasis on day care and minimal intervention surgery, these patients will constitute the majority of clients in the future.

For most patients illness and disease is 'a moment of truth'. Even a hernia can bring into focus some aspect of that person's life which he had never thought about. Most illness brings with it a kind of loss: a loss of health, of an organ, of time, of relationships, of mobility or life-style. This generally concerns both the patients or clients, and their families, friends and others who are significant in their lives. Most of us go through life with an attitude of 'it won't happen to me' and, when it does, the moment of truth can be quite shattering. It need not be a big blow, like an accident or cancer. Having your bunions done is just as often a trigger for facing that 'it *has* happened to me'. An external event is the vehicle for internal searching and adjustment. When, as a nurse, you show a patient that you are aware of these possibilities and take them into account whilst discussing them, your style becomes 'emotional' and the patient responds favourably.

In this helping, the three constant components are therefore the helper, the client and the relationship between them.

The helper

As the discipline of counselling grew, it became clear that those who use the skills need to have certain attitudes and show certain recognized skills. These are now generally summed up as genuineness, warmth and empathy, though not necessarily always in this order. The order matters less because these skills and attitudes overlap and interact. Some difficulty has been encountered, particularly with empathy, which is considered both an attitude and a skill. These three elements will be considered below. Before this, I would like to concentrate on some attitudes that helpers bring to any relationship and any helping. They have to be there before helping is even considered. These are not the only attitudes needed: others may also be there, but they are not listed here. Readers may want to be aware of other attitudes which they recognize in themselves and others.

Attitudes

Attentiveness Asking a client 'how are you?' when you are unwilling to hear the answer can be awkward as well as painful. We all know how diminished we can feel when we are ignored by someone we know or care about.

You can be talking with someone while thinking of the train you will be missing, what shopping to get on the way home, or all the jobs you have not done yet. This happens easily when the client's story is laboriously told, or seemingly boring, or, indeed, you simply do not want to be with this person at this time.

Attentiveness means being present in both body and spirit. The quality of the presence is what matters most. Clearly, in any interaction there will be distractions on both sides. It matters that your self-awareness is acute enough to pick these distractions up and that your values are such that you know – at least in general terms – what you will be doing about your distractions.

Attentiveness is a kind of willingness to be there, to present a certain emptiness to the other person to accept anything that he or she may bring, and a willingness to share yourself, your time, and your skills and gifts.

Carkhuff (1987, p. 15) calls attending a 'pre-helping skill' for the phases of helping. For him, attending is a skill that enables clients to become involved. When attentiveness is considered from the point of view of an attitude, it becomes clear that basic attentiveness leads to the development of a process, a relationship and, hopefully, the self-help skills that make for more resourceful living.

Non-judgemental attitude   A non-judgemental attitude is such a basic requirement that it runs the risk of being taken for granted. Being non-judgemental does not mean 'anything goes', or that no judgements can be made at all. Indeed, you have to make judgements all the time to live. When a distinction is made between the attitude and the skill of judgement, it may be easier to see that it is the attitude which matters here.

Carkhuff (1987, p. 78) says that this attitude demands from helpers a suspension of premature solutions, of personal attitudes, and of personal values. These last two items constitute the attitude as described here, whereas the first refers more clearly to the skill of judging.

Included in a non-judgemental attitude is the notion of respect. This means that the person with you is accepted for what he or she is. This is not restricted to helping and counselling, but is an attitude which you have to everyone. As this is a basic moral principle, there is a strong emphasis on this being a pre-requisite for all interaction, especially one done from a sense of wanting to help.

Suspending your judgement may occasionally lead to conflict. This is particularly so when strong views abound, or when the subject under discussion is one in which you have religious, political or professional interests. Can you then leave these behind and be an impartial helper? Perhaps yes, perhaps no. It depends entirely on your experience at handling such situations, and what your values or attitudes are. If there is likely to be conflict, the best way may be to declare your interests and negotiate with the client as to whether you are the best person to help. Helping should never be done at the expense of your conscience. But clearly, helping is not imposing your solutions, attitudes and values.

Being hopeful   Many helping situations are created because of hopelessness and helplessness in clients. The 'moment of truth' may have shown up something that presents itself as a closed door, an impossibly high mountain, or a chasm so deep that it appears impossible to get to the other side. A basic attitude of hopefulness by helpers is therefore essential. Without such an attitude, you might never undertake helping and counselling – and indeed, nursing.

Being hopeful is radically different from being optimistic. An optimist seizes opportunities and looks for short-term gains. Being hopeful means telling the person with you that you believe in them, that you believe in their intrinsic worth and goodness, and that you convey to them that they are worth your effort, time and skilled care.

When you respect someone you are in effect showing them that you are taking very seriously what you are hearing in terms of worthlessness, fear, hopelessness and inability to move forward. But you are at the same time indicating *that this is not all that there is*. As a helper and counsellor you believe in a life after this crisis, problem, illness, or whatever has created the present impasse. Human experience of life has shown that people can and do move on and change. It is this belief which you cling to and by your attitude convey to the persons you are concerned with. This does mean that you believe this first of all about yourself. If you do not have such a basic conviction, then you are less able to help others to be hopeful.

An attitude of hopefulness does not say, 'There, there, don't fret, tomorrow everything will be fine', because it may not be. Being hopeful does mean, though, that you believe in the capacity of human beings to change, by whatever powers they name.

Being supportive   If you are hopeful by attitude, then you are probably also supportive. It would be ironic to convey hopefulness and then not be supportive.

The attitude of supportiveness means that it is necessary to form a relationship with someone for the duration of the problem. This is probably a short time in nursing settings where most helping is done around a one-off problem. When it means a longer span of time, then clearly there is more emphasis on the relationship and its therapeutic role. This can then also be called 'getting involved'.

If you want to help others, you cannot help but be involved. Merely by showing interest in someone you become involved. When you are attentive to someone you are involved, because two human beings relate. You need to be involved with others in order to stay human. The 'getting involved' which people fear means starting a relationship and then finding that more is asked of you than you can give. What do you then do?

Being supportive does not mean overstepping every boundary. I sometimes have an image of helpers being like amoeba, going after every bit of helping possible, changing shape constantly to accommodate yet one more request. This is not necessarily self-forgetfulness, but a selfish search for filling up an insatiable desire to be needed. Such people cannot be supportive to others because they are too much in need of support themselves.

When you are supportive you still have your own boundaries. If you have an attitude of attentiveness, of being non-judgemental and hopeful, then you *are* supportive already. Like so much else in counselling, you have to be supportive to yourself first, before you can be supportive to others. When you know how to be supportive to yourself – when you know your boundaries – then you are already supportive to others.

These basic helper attitudes are not exclusive, but I believe that they need to be present in some form or another in people who want to help others. They are included in the core conditions of genuineness, warmth and empathy, which will now be considered. The emphasis there is, however, more on the skills than the attitudes.

'Core conditions'

Genuineness Egan (1994, p. 55) calls his section on genuineness 'Beyond professionalism and phoneyness'. This makes it quite clear that here, too, there is both an attitude and a skill involved.

Genuineness, or congruence, is something that is learnt over many years. As you become more and more congruent, so you become more effective in helping. This is what Rogers (1961) (see Chapter 1) had come to see, too: if he tried to be 'the counsellor' and disregarded persistent feelings between himself and a client, the relationship suffered. When he learned to be more and more himself as one person with another, then he was or became congruent and this was experienced as trustworthy.

Mearns and Thorne (1988, p. 76) say that 'congruence is a state of being of the counsellor throughout her contact with the client, and as such it usually goes unnoticed'. As with all the attitudes mentioned so far, genuineness is not particularly obvious when present, but when it is not there the clients are aware of the lack.

For congruence to have an impact on the relationship between counsellor and client the latter must perceive the counsellor as being congruent. It does not matter how authentic the counsellor is being: if the client perceives her as duplicit or insincere the therapeutic impact of congruence will be substantially lost. (Mearns and Thorne, 1988, p. 76)

Genuineness means, basically, that what you think and what you say is the same. If clients really get on your nerves, for whatever reason, and you assure them that they have your undivided attention, then there is clearly a credibility gap. In one way or another clients will perceive this. With a measure of self-awareness you will be able to notice what is happening and this allows you to change.

Genuineness does not mean that you 'should blurt out whatever feelings (you) are experiencing in an effort to be congruent' (Bayne et al., 1994, p. 27), such as telling your clients that they get on your nerves. Indeed, it is not they who do something to you, but you who are experiencing certain feelings towards them. There may be very good reasons for such feelings. The attitudes and skills of counselling demand in such a situation a 'need to make careful decisions about how much to share in the moment, and how much should be considered later and elsewhere' (Bayne et al., 1994, p. 27).

As often, it is Egan (1994, p. 55) who details very simply what genuineness consists of. He lists four aspects:

Do not overemphasize the helping role.
Be spontaneous.
Avoid defensiveness.
Be open.

Perhaps these headings indicate that the more human, 'ordinary' and unaffected you can be with your clients, the more your helping is real and effective.

Patient:	How do you think I am getting on?
Nurse:	Very well, as far as I can see. This fracture is healing well.
Patient:	So you think I can leave soon and get back to my own life?
Nurse:	It will be a fortnight yet before you get your crutches, but then you should be well on your way.
Patient:	I just wish I had died in that accident.
Nurse:	What makes you say that?
Patient:	I just wish I were dead.
Nurse:	I am not sure what to think or say now. I am picking up two very different messages: one that you want to live and one that you wish you were dead.

Patient: I want to live, but I also want to be gone and be with B. Can you understand this?

Nurse: Not really... but I would like to try. Perhaps you could tell me a bit more of what you mean.

This interaction shows many of the attitudes and skills needed for counselling. When concentrating on genuineness or congruence, it is clear that this helper did not put on a mask of 'counsellor' by trying to understand a very complex response, possibly twisting her mind into contortions and still sounding unconvincing in a reply. Instead, just as in any normal conversation, the helper answered by saying that she was not sure what to think in the first reply, and in the second reply she clearly said that she did not understand what the patient was hinting at.

In a summary of what congruence is, Mearns and Thorne (1988, p. 83) say that the skill of congruence is a response to the client's expressions; this response has to be relevant to the client; the response is either to something persistent or striking which the client notices. In the above example it can be seen that the helper responds to (a) a double message and (b) a request for understanding, both of which are striking; and the helper's response is relevant to the client in that it shows up the double message he gives.

Warmth   This component of helping has been described in many ways: 'non-possessive warmth' and 'unconditional positive regard' are perhaps the best known.

Rogers (1980, p. 310) cites a study done with teachers and students in which it was found that teachers who got the best out of their students had high levels of self-regard, disclosed themselves to the students, responded to their feelings and ideas, gave them praise, and 'lectured' less often.

The teachers had a high regard for themselves. They did not show off, but somehow knew their place in the world and felt at home in it. Therefore they could share, listen, praise, and not feel threatened or throw their weight around. They worked hard and played hard. They came across as genuine people.

Being warm does not necessarily mean being effusive, particularly if this is not your style or normal way of behaving. It means first and foremost respecting the other person and what that person is and stands for. It is also possible that, because of unconditional positive regard, you come to like or even love a person with whom you may at first not have felt much rapport. This is not easy. We have all said to others, 'Be a dear and get me. . .', and so made our love conditional. All too often the love encountered in families is conditional and we have grown up with this and perpetuate it. It may therefore take a conscious effort to be different.

According to Mearns and Thorne (1988, p. 59) unconditional positive regard is

the label given to the fundamental attitude of the person-centred coun-sellor towards the client. The counsellor who holds this attitude deeply values the humanity of her client and is not deflected in that valuing by any particular client behaviours. The attitude manifests itself in the counsellor's consistent acceptance of and enduring warmth towards her client.

These authors call warmth an attitude, which indeed it is, but the skills they describe show that it is also more than just an attitude. Indeed, Mearns and Thorne (1988, p. 59) show that warmth (or unconditional positive regard) is more often a response to attitudes held by clients. These attitudes are described as a 'self-defeating cycle', with the client adopting a stance of

'I behave more and more defensively
That keeps other people away
Nobody cares for me'.

When people are ill, they are vulnerable, and that leads very easily and quickly to feelings of being useless, sad and fearful. In such a position it is not easy to be positive or sure about what decisions to make. This is why patients need much reassurance; or so we imagine.

What patients may need much more than reassurance may be this unconditional positive regard. Reassurance can too easily be a glib answer, given from a position of superior knowledge, with many assumptions between patient and nurse not voiced and perhaps deliberately not acknowledged. When you use the skills of this component of helping, you may therefore be much nearer the 'real thing'.

Patient:	I feel so awful having given you all this work.
Nurse:	It's not been a chore to me.
Patient:	It's difficult to accept having to be looked after.
Nurse:	I can understand that, but you also give me something when I care for you.
Patient:	Really. . .?

Nurse:	Just being in contact with you makes me feel pleased to be a nurse.
Patient:	I find this difficult to believe under the circumstances.
Nurse:	There! (giving the patient a kiss and a hug)

There are many degrees of warmth between a simple touch and a bear hug; between a smile and a phrase perhaps repeated often to show that you mean what you say. It is not *your* warmth which clients need to see; rather they need to experience warmth that is adequate to their needs.

Empathy   Rogers (1957) was the first to use the term empathy as part of therapy. In 1980 he wrote what has become a definitive statement about empathy:

It means entering the private perceptual world of the other and becoming thoroughly at home in it. It involves being sensitive, moment by moment, to the changing felt meanings which flow in this person, to the fear or rage or tenderness or confusion or whatever that he or she is experiencing. It means temporarily living in the other's life, moving about in it delicately without making judgements. (Rogers, 1980, p. 142)

A short and cogent definition of empathy has been written by Kalisch (1971): 'Empathy is the ability to perceive accurately the feelings of another person and to communicate this understanding to him (or her)'. This definition points to the two-way nature of empathy: understanding the other person, and reflecting that understanding to him or her. It is not enough for the helper to understand a client, the client also needs to be helped by this understanding.

Mayeroff (1971, p. 30) describes this understanding in a philosophical way, and from the point of view of caring:

To care for another person I must be able to understand him and his world as if I were inside it. I must be able to see, as it were, with his eyes what his world is like to him and how he sees himself. Instead of merely looking at him in a detached way from outside, as if he were a specimen, I must be able to be with him in his world, 'going' into his world in order to sense from 'inside' what life is like for him, what he is striving to be, and what he requires to grow.

Some people have described this capacity of understanding as walking in the other's shoes. I am not happy about this metaphor, because walking in the other's shoes implies pushing him or her out of his or her own shoes. It implies a taking over of the other's life. I think that it is more accurate to say that what is implied is an understanding of what it feels like for the other to be in his or her own shoes. In this way we are in the client's world, sensing from the inside what his or her life is like.

Empathy or sympathy? The following allegory may highlight the difference between empathy and sympathy.

A person has fallen into a ditch, and is unable to get out of it. A *sympathetic* person comes along, sees the victim, goes to him and lies in the ditch with him, and both talk of this terrible misadventure and of other similar ones they had both experienced in the past. An *unsympathetic* person comes along the road, sees the person lying there and shouts to him 'Don't just lie there, pull yourself together, do something!' But the victim has broken bones, and he cannot move, and the helper neither sees nor hears what the victim is saying because she is standing too far away. An *empathic* person who comes that way climbs down to the victim and gives what first aid is necessary. Then she listens to what the victim has to say, how the accident happened, what led up to it, and what he now feels and experiences. This helper is completely present, but figuratively she has one foot on the bank, the firm ground. This eventually enables her to help the victim get out of the ditch on to his own legs, and to the way he wants to go, the way that is right for him.

To begin with, many helping situations need some practical help: information, the right form to fill in or a telephone call. Equally, to begin with, a person may 'just' need to talk and be heard. Anyone shocked and numbed needs nurturing, not counselling. 'Tea and sympathy' is not such a bad thing, as long as you keep one foot on the firm ground and change to empathy when the moment is right.

Daniel (1984) distinguishes empathy from sympathy by saying that the prefix 'em' corresponds to 'en' or 'in', as in insight or intuition, whereas in sympathy the prefix 'sym' corresponds to 'syn' or 'like'. Empathy, she says, 'is an intuitive leap of mind and feeling which encompasses all the aspects and the condition of the sufferer'. Empathy is deeper than sympathy, because it goes 'in' and uses imagination. Sympathy, being 'like', cannot make that leap of 'sensitive receptivity to the suffering of another' because it is too much tied to the self. Sympathy compares with another; insight is achieved only with empathy.

Being empathic

What then is empathy? How is it expressed, recognized, communicated?

One of the difficulties with empathy is clearly that Rogers (1980) saw it as 'a way of being', whereas others saw it in terms of skills. Skills are measurable and teachable, whereas the 'way of being' eludes the researcher's pad. In effect, both are necessary and one without the other is rather hollow.

Taylor (1972, p. 243) tells of a story where empathy was expressed in action:

A colleague has recently described to me an occasion when a West Indian woman in a London flat was told of her husband's death in a street accident. The shock of the grief stunned her like a blow, she sank into a corner of the sofa and sat there rigid and unhearing. For a long time her terrible tranced look continued to embarrass the family, friends and officials who came and went. Then the schoolteacher of one of her children, an Englishwoman, called, and seeing how things were, went and sat beside her. Without a word she threw an arm around the tight shoulders, clasping them with her full strength. The white cheek was thrust hard against the brown. Then as the unrelenting pain seeped through to her, the newcomer's tears began to flow, falling on their two hands linked in the woman's lap. For a long time that is all that was happening. And then at last the West Indian woman started to sob. Still not a word was spoken and after a little while the visitor got up and went, leaving her contribution to help the family meet its immediate needs.

By entering caringly into the world of another, some people communicate their understanding through action; others might use words; still others might use both.

As with the other components of helping, we are not usually aware that they are being used, but when they are not present we feel disappointed and not helped. The skills of empathy are now described and detailed.

Truax (1961) had established a comprehensive eight-point scale of empathy. Egan (1994) speaks of two levels of empathy. The first, which he calls basic empathy, is understood to be a communication skill. The helper responds to the words spoken and reflects them: there is an initial communication of a basic understanding, as in this dialogue between patient and nurse.

Patient: I feel really terrible today, worse than yesterday.
Nurse: You feel worse today?

The *words* are repeated, or reflected. This is the basic act of empathy: the helper shows that the client is heard. The helper acknowledges that hearing by going no further than the client, and staying at the same level as the client. Responding to the words spoken is the initial essential step in helping.

Patient: I feel really terrible today, worse than yesterday.
Nurse: Don't worry, these things take time.

This nurse has heard the words, and is responding to the implication, but inappropriately and not empathically. After such an interaction there is nothing more for a client to say. The nurse has indicated that she or he does not want to hear anything further. This is clearly an unempathic remark.

The first simple response to the words shows that the helper wants to hear more. This nurse is ready to listen. In the image of the story, this nurse starts to climb down to the victim and makes the first move towards him. Responding to the words spoken is, in Egan's (1994, p. 106) terms, 'basic empathy'. The information that the client gives is received by the helper who, in responding with the same words as those used by the client, shows that she or he has heard. At the same time this is also a check that the information is correct. Essentially the skill of reflecting (see Chapter 8) is used here.

This basic level may be used initially, in the first few exchanges of a conversation. When enough information has been given and received, the helper should then move on to the second stage of advanced empathy. There is less reflection of words, but more of feelings, of implied behaviours, and of underlying trends. At this level, intuition and 'hunches' play a role, and there is some interpretation going on. This second, deeper level of empathy picks out the unspoken feeling or reason behind what is said.

Patient: I feel terrible today, worse than yesterday.
Nurse: You sound dejected at feeling worse today.

Both levels of empathy are necessary. In most interactions there is a certain amount of initial information giving and receiving before the conversation can go deeper. The helper who listens well will have taken any such cues from the client, and not have offered them unsolicited.

Recognizing two levels of empathy is useful for training and learning purposes. Once you use them they will come quite spontaneously. It is important to realize that in any interaction both levels of empathy are generally used side by side. To begin with, the basic level is used most, going on to the advanced level gradually. If only the basic level is used, a client may still reach a goal, but more slowly and laboriously, or the conversation may grind to a halt, because no *helping* is actually done, even though reflection may take place.

Even when using advanced empathy it is helpful to come back to simple reflection and to basic empathy. The two levels need to be used side by side. A basic level response is often necessary to check something out: 'Is that the right feeling?' or 'Was that what you said?' or 'Am I right in thinking. . .?'

Patient:	I can't use the time the way I would like to. That's the worst part.
Nurse:	Is that what is bothering you?
Patient:	Yes, the fact that I can't use the time profitably. . . I suppose basically I am not a man of action.
Nurse:	You are not a man of action?
Patient:	No. That surprises you?
Nurse:	It does surprise me.
Patient:	I am . . . what am I?

On the level of skill, this is perhaps more an example of genuineness than empathy. It shows good basic empathy and, without many words, this interaction perhaps enabled the patient to do some further thinking about his present position and illness.

Empathy is a very basic element in helping, but it cannot be separated from genuineness and warmth. All the components discussed so far are necessary – as are all those that will be discussed in later chapters. Perhaps the discussion so far has highlighted only that helping is a whole. You have to think in terms of the book, not the individual chapters.

The client

The focus of helping is clearly the client. It must be kept in mind, though, that both client and helper gain from this work of helping, and that therefore there is a sharing going on which is not necessarily equal, but is real for both people.

A person may be a 'client' – in the sense of receiving particular counselling help – for only a very short time; for several short episodes; or for regular help. Thus it is difficult to paint a picture of a 'typical' client. I will consider here only patients as clients, fully aware that in the wider context of this book I would also include colleagues and friends under the heading of 'client'.

The various models for helping point out that feelings play a major part in helping. Feelings are often either ruling a person or cannot be accessed because of long suppression through conditioning. Discerning what are the present and underlying feelings in the story a client presents is therefore very important in the helping process. It may be useful to consider some of the more common feelings encountered by patients in some detail. While these feelings are described here as belonging to patients, it is quite clear that they also at times belong to nurses, carers and helpers of every kind. We are all at the same time unique and 'Everyman' and 'Everywoman'.

Fear

A person's reactions to most situations of threat to individuality, maturity or survival is either fear or anger.

If we were to set down in order of importance the diverse feelings of our patients, fear would lead them all. Fear, perhaps the most powerful of all emotions, can give rise to behaviour over which patients have little or no control (Burton, 1979, p. 13).

Fear is a remarkably strong influence in most people's lives. Faced with anything unusual, we are afraid, and not just a little. When we are afraid, we generally fear 'the worst'. The woman who has discovered a lump in her breast fears 'the worst', that it is cancer, and her mind leaps to the thought 'death'. The person in an accident who has badly broken a leg fears 'the worst', that the leg might have to be amputated, and the mind leaps to 'my life ruined'.

Once the identity is threatened, we can become quite unable to handle simple, otherwise ordinary, situations. We believe that everything is working against us. Fear creates fear, and a spiral of fear leads to irrational behaviour. 'The only thing we have to fear is fear itself', said President Roosevelt, and not unjustly.

Fear tends to be a threat of danger to survival:

I won't make it.

This is a fear of physical survival, but it is also a fear of emotional survival.

I won't come through this operation.
I am no good as a woman any more.
I fear pain, therefore I won't have this test.
I feel I can't cope; don't ask me to help.
I don't trust myself; I always make a fool of myself.

Gilbert (1989) has described the basic mechanisms of defence as a 'go–stop process'. Fear leads more often to 'stop', and anger to 'go'. The behaviours and reactions arising out of fear are the helplessness and hopelessness so often seen in patients, and the paralysing inability to take any rational decision.

Anger and hostility

Anger is a common reaction to attack, be this attack by another person or an illness. What cannot be handled calmly and assertively gets the angry treatment.

It has been said that the best defence is a good offence. People lash out at others before they can be attacked themselves. Burton (1979, p. 83) says that a fight reaction may be exactly what the words imply: hostile, resentful, belligerent ways which may or may not involve physical activity. Gilbert (1989) calls this the 'go' part of the process of defence, and nurses know it as 'fight': the time when the adrenalin rises.

Physical aggression may lead to injury, as it is meant to 'kill' the threat. In fact, few people recognize how hostile they can be. Nurses are often the first in line of an attack by a patient, but doctors, radiographers, porters and ambulance crews are all liable to be attacked. Such behaviour is normal when it is seen as part of a pattern of adjustment. When the anger has blown over, such a person will often recognize where it came from, and will realize that the extent of personal involvement is not only the other's fault.

Nurses need to recognize that their professional standards may not be the same as other people's standards, and what they regard as a small matter and part of their work may spark off quite unexpected, hostile reactions in others.

Nurses who are on the receiving end of verbal or physical attacks may take it personally and see it as a slight on their care-giving. This is not so. It is the client's problem: it is their fear, their uncertainty, their anger and their inability to cope. Physical attacks should never be condoned, but helping a person through anger is a challenge to anyone.

Shock

I collapsed at work on the Monday morning. I drove to work, walked across the car park and my left leg buckled underneath me; I couldn't stand. They took me to hospital and they did lots and lots of tests.

They got Dr N to see me, and he said, 'Oh yes!', all bright and cheerful, 'you've got a tumour on the brain'. Well, that was a terrible shock. (Tschudin, 1981)

This patient had difficulty in believing that her left leg indicated that she had a tumour in her head. It would have been easier to believe that there was something wrong with her legs.

Another patient told of

how after some weeks of feeling unwell she woke up one morning realizing that her left side was paralysed. She simply closed her eyes again and went to sleep for a few more hours.

Kate was a paediatrician and the wife of Charles who had just been to outpatients to have metastases from a melanoma confirmed. Kate and Charles lived separately but often spoke on the phone. Before Charles phoned Kate with his news he phoned a few friends to ask them whether he should have the proposed treatment or go for complementary therapy. When he phoned Kate he told her he would not have an operation but go to a clinic known to him. Kate was so shocked by this decision that she rang all the friends she expected Charles had contacted to find out exactly what they had told him. In her shock she needed to have others to blame.

The instinctive reaction to any bad news often is 'Oh no!' The characteristic of shock is denial of what has happened: it can't be true; this can't be happening to me.

The way in which this shock is expressed varies greatly. The patient who simply went to sleep again said that normally she never slept in. It may be a state of complete disorientation, or it may be the opposite: carrying on as if nothing had happened. In shock an abnormal reaction to an abnormal situation seems to be normal.

Like physical shock, emotional shock will change and wear off. And, as with physical shock, a person who is emotionally shocked needs gentle handling. A shocked person will probably not hear much of what is said, but will often respond to touch. When people are 'frozen', the warmth of close contact can be the most appropriate way to help them to come to the reality of the present. The 'unfreezing' happens when the person begins to talk. And then, like melting ice, the talking may be fast and abundant.

Shock is a way of handling bad news of any kind. 'Tea and sympathy' has long been considered a standard remedy for this type of situation. While it has its limitations, this dictum has some validity.

Disbelief

In the process of adjustment to anything unexpected, such as illness, accidents, bereavement or loss of any kind, there is always a time of denial. The person who had a leg amputated still feels it clearly; the bereaved person still feels the missing partner in bed; when you have had something stolen you can still touch it. This is a normal phenomenon and a way in which the psyche or mind comes to terms with what has happened. To cut oneself off all at once from something that had been essential to life seems impossible; therefore a time of disbelief is like a process of gradually letting go of what is now no longer there.

A mentally healthy person will be able to see this as a stage and work through it, going from an instinctive disbelief to accepting and believing that it *did* happen, or *is* happening.

When disbelief turns into a more permanent mechanism of defence, then it becomes a denial of the past and the present. The patient is denying having cancer and tells her relatives and friends that the surgeon just took the breast off as a pre-caution. To counter such a statement with 'But you do have cancer' is not helpful because in that person's make-believe world there is no such thing as cancer. To see it as a coping or defence mechanism would be more realistic, and could form the basis for giving help.

Misunderstanding

A very common defence mechanism of patients is that of not hearing what has been said, or hearing only what they want to hear or can cope with.

The doctor that I'm under, he's told me that he can cure me. At the start when I came down to London, they found that I had a small pancreas in the back of my head, and the fluid couldn't drain out at the other side and had stopped working. So they fitted a small pump and a tube that goes to a bag at the side of my bladder, that pumps it through so that the bladder is not overloaded. They also found this tumour which they said they can't get out by a normal operation, as under the knife. It could cause me to be paralysed, or could cause blindness, or something like that. But the doctor I am under now, he said they can cure it. They are treating my spine as well now so that the tumour separates the cells going down to my nervous system which could make me paralysed. So they can cure it now. (Tschudin, 1981)

This tale, from a taped interview, shows that the patient heard only what he could grasp. Some knowledge, some apprehension, an old wives' tale or two picked up somewhere, new and unusual surroundings, and the recipe for misunderstanding is complete.

Anyone who has ever asked for street directions will appreciate the problem. You may correctly hear the first direction or two, but then you get lost in right and left turns. You cannot cope with too much information when you are under stress, even the relatively minor stress of being lost in the street.

A man may be nervous about seeing a doctor in the first place. He may have some questions to ask, but the doctor talks first. The doctor will probably use some medical terms of which the patient is unsure, but the patient is unwilling to appear ignorant. The apprehensive patient may have forgotten to switch his hearing aid on. Later, the doctor may say the same to the patient's wife, but when the patient and his wife compare what they have heard or understand, their stories differ.

It may only be a question of clarifying a word or technical term, or explaining a test or operation more fully. But, like denial, misunderstanding may have become a way of life and a permanent mechanism. The skill of helping is to see the difference and deal with it empathically.

Guilt

While anger blames the 'other', whatever or whoever it may be, guilt blames the self. Guilt is a complex of feelings because there are several different aspects to it which are often confused or misunderstood. Dryden (1994, p. 2) describes three different conditions under which guilt occurs:

1. There is guilt when a person feels that a moral code, principle, standard or value has been broken. When a dogmatic attitude is then used to interpret this act, guilt will result.
2. There is guilt when a person focuses on the consequences of what has been done or not done. This happens in particular when another person has been hurt in some way.
3. There is guilt when there is a dogmatic attitude towards the self which focuses on who or what the person is in general.

The first two types of guilt arise from some action or episode, hence Dryden calls this 'episodic guilt'. Dryden calls the third type 'existential guilt'.

Given these conditions when guilt arises, Dryden then distinguishes two kinds of guilt:

1. Guilt as an unconstructive emotion.
2. Guilt as constructive remorse.

The difference between these two types seems to lie in the dogmatic attitude that many people apply. This seems to stem from a sense of excessive responsibility or from irrational beliefs. Feelings of guilt and self-blame are very common in patients with cancer, or in their partners (King, 1984). Guilt can also exist when a patient believes that he or she is infectious or 'dirty'. Such patients may reject help of any kind, as they believe or imagine themselves to be outcast and beyond the reach of help. These are clear examples of existential guilt and so-called irrational feelings.

Dryden (1994) focuses his book on overcoming guilt, and shows how to help people to see the difference between constructive and unconstructive elements in their feelings. The constructive remorse leads to change and restitution (if necessary) and thus to a healthier way of life.

Constructive remorse, concern and sadness constitute what can be called the 'compassionate self'. Those who develop a compassionate attitude towards themselves for their wrongdoings are more likely to experience remorse when they break their moral code than guilt. (Dryden, 1994, p. 19)

Some would argue that today people are more indulgent and therefore guilt is taken less seriously. This may apply perhaps to younger people. Older people have grown up in a culture that helped to create a climate of excessive guilt, which is therefore encountered regularly in people who are at critical stages in their life. If it is possible then to help them to see what may be irrational, unconstructive or excessive, we may have helped them in the most constructive way.

Shame

Shame is a kind of uncovering or appearing naked. According to Erikson (1964), shame can begin to appear in a child as early as the second year of life. During that year, a child becomes capable of independent action. If a child fails at such actions, shame and doubt develop.

Shame is first of all an uncovering of ourselves to ourselves: 'A shame experience might be defined as an acute emotional awareness of a failure to *be* in some way' (Egan, 1994, p. 148). The inadequacy is there, but is unrecognized until, because of some remark, happening or association, the inadequacy – the shame – is consciously recognized.

The area most often associated with shame is sexuality. We learn early to keep that subject under the duvet. Many people connect illness, particularly of the sexual organs, with wrong-doing in the past, with punishment, and with sin and guilt. They are ashamed of themselves for having such a disease. They imagine that the world around them will now find out or know about their wrongdoing. They feel that they should not or could not talk about their illness.

Such people suffer guilt in silence, giving thoughts, feelings and a negative imagination a stranglehold over them. It is all too easy to brush feelings of shame aside. 'Self-blame typically occurs in the absence of any other known or acceptable explanation' (King, 1984). Sometimes a simple explanation of anatomy can help a patient to see an illness or disease in perspective, where before no meaningful connection was possible.

Feelings of shame can and need to be recognized and acknowledged. When recognized, they can become valuable tools for growth and development.

Regression

Attitudes towards illness and people who can help one to get better are learnt in childhood. When a person becomes seriously ill, this attitude can be triggered into action and a grown person can behave like a child. Some children seek attention by 'being good' and submissive; others gain what they need by crying, moaning or complaining (Altschul and Sinclair, 1981, p. 152).

Mathews (1962) notes that

adult hospital patients, because of their fright and insecurity in the situation, regress to a child-like dependency and continuously seek reassurance. At the same time, however, this dependent status sets up a deep conflict within patients in their attempts to maintain the self-image as an adult. Patients react strongly against threats to their individuality, maturity and adulthood.

Nurses who are aware of such behaviour are more likely to deal sympathetically with patients, rather than dismissing it or playing the game with them. The notion of a partnership addresses the adult behaviour in patients, and this in itself can be therapeutic because it allows them to be, and be seen as, responsible.

The helping relationship

The helping relationship has been written about, studied and analysed by a great many writers, and yet it is something that is essentially indefinable. In the same way that two people can be in love with each other and their friends wonder whatever it is that attracts them, so a relationship between a helper and client can be effective and therapeutic, although this may not be possible between the same helper and another patient.

There are some elements about relationships that should be mentioned here. Later chapters will deal with the skills of helping, which are at the same time skills of relating.

All helping and counselling is done within a relationship. In nursing, a relationship is already given, in that every patient is looked after by at least one, if not more, nurses. The way you use that relationship is therefore of paramount importance.

Be aware for a moment how your contact with a patient starts:

1. The patient is sick; the nurse is healthy.
2. The patient is needy; the nurse can fulfil the need.
3. The patient has only the nurse to relate to; the nurse has other patients and colleagues if she or he needs a break.
4. The patient is dependent; the nurse has power.
5. The patient is lying down; the nurse is standing over him or her.
6. The patient may have needs of intimate bodily care; the nurse, a stranger, gives it without question.

This list makes it quite clear that the relationship between a nurse and patient is basically a very unequal one: one has and the other has not. This is true of many other situations but the inequality is often reduced, in that the one who needs a service pays for it. The two partners thus become more equal. In nursing, this is impossible.

The relationship is also very human, and there are thus many possibilities of feelings of dependency and counter-dependency, trust and mistrust, transference and counter-transference (see Chapter 12) between patients and nurses which may help or hinder, be conscious or uncounscious. Simply being aware of the possibility is often helpful. When these elements do present themselves, they can be acknowledged and faced.

Hierarchies still exist very strongly in nursing, at least here in Britain, despite many efforts at reducing this. Relationships based on power and authority are not readily tolerated any longer, but it is not easy to change to other systems of relating when the culture has not generally changed. It is therefore quite difficult to switch to a different style of relating when counselling. This is perhaps when the essential attitudes of helpers are particularly called upon, and when respecting the person of the client is a fundamental need.

Salvage (1990) has pointed out that the 'new nursing' is based on partnership. Such a relationship is creative for both parties. It is also one that challenges. Given the unequal starting point of the nurse–patient relationship, partnership has to be worked on and established by negotiation.

In this kind of helping relationship there is no clear distinction between physical and psychological care. One generally leads to the other, and they overlap and interact. A diabetic patient on a special diet needs advice about it; but she may also need to discuss fears about her future and her children's future; what this disease means to her; or any other aspect of life that is important to her. The challenge to the nurse is to deal with the *person*, not just her problems.

Like a story, relationships have a beginning, a middle and an end. And like learning to write, making, keeping and ending helping relationships have to be learned. It is not just a question of using the right social or communication skills; it is a question of helping another person by and through *being with* that person.

Because much of the helping done in nursing is one-off and directly concerned with a specific problem, there is not the same need to build and negotiate the relationship. But however short or long, superficial or deep the meeting between two people is, such meetings are for helping. It is therefore essential that the client should benefit. Murgatroyd (1985, p. 34) details some features of helping that are valued by those who have been helped:

1. They have been encouraged to increase their self-understanding.
2. They have been helped to see how similar they are to others, particularly if they have felt out of touch with others beforehand. This can be important for patients who feel that nobody understands what they are going through, perhaps when a diagnosis has not been clearly established.
3. They feel that they have been understood, accepted and responded to genuinely by their helpers.

4. They have been made aware of how others see them.
5. They have been encouraged to talk about themselves, to be assertive and immediate in their reactions.
6. They have appreciated the openness and warmth of their helpers, even when the helpers confronted them.
7. They have most respected those helpers who are themselves and do not play the role of helper when they work with clients.
8. They have appreciated the opportunity to share and divulge inner thoughts and feelings in a safe and neutral atmosphere.

'Rogers argued that the relationship that develops between counsellor and client is the most significant agent of change, not the counsellor's repertoire of techniques' (Bayne et al., 1994, p. 31). Bayne and colleagues consider this a controversial point of view. Rogers, however, maintained this position because he believed that people have within them the personal resources needed for change, which cannot be supplied from outside. As long as clients are understood empathically by someone trustworthy and non-judgemental, clients can deal with negative conditioning. Rogers also believed that the counselling relationship should be an egalitarian one, with power being shared between client and counsellor.

Because the text of a book is linear, it is almost impossible to demonstrate the dynamic of the relationship. What therefore happens in actual life is possibly very different from the description here. The work being done by client and helper changes and the emphasis of the work being done therefore also changes. This is clear in that, to begin with, the helper's skills are paramount for the formation of a relationship and to get the helping process underway. Towards the end of the process it is the clients who do most of the work with their inherent skills called forth and new ones developed sufficiently to function in a 'skilled' way.

Different authors have described this shift in emphasis and dynamic in different ways. I will do this in a sequential way in the following chapters by considering the differing skills needed by helper and client. It must be clear, though, that without the skills of the helper, clients cannot develop their skills; and the helper's skills are valid only because the clients need them. Thus there is another element of interdependence, and another reason for demonstrating that, indeed, the counselling relationship is an egalitarian one.

The contexts in which counselling can and does happen are as varied as the people concerned. Hospitals and sickrooms can be disturbing places. The symbols of operations, of cutting and hurting, submitting to people who invade the body or stick needles into it and take bits out of it are very powerful at all levels of care. It need not only be the obvious operations, investigations and treatments that call for counselling help; sometimes the silent diseases of fear and guilt also need 'the sharp compassion of the healer's art' (Eliot, 1944, p. 29). The healers here are all those who enter into a relationship with another person.

CHAPTER SEVEN

Helping skills: attending

....

Attending

Have you ever experienced talking to someone and that other person looked at someone else, tried to pull a thread from a sleeve, or did not give you an answer when you expected one? If so, you know what not attending is about. You also know how painful this can be as you feel devalued and not important.

Attending is very simple and at the same time very demanding. It means a 'being there' in body and mind. Carkhuff (1987) comes back to attending again and again when describing his model.

Attending means that you orient yourself towards the client. You are with this person. You convey to your client that you are here just for her or him at this moment. You turn off your bleep or telephone. You ensure, as far as possible, that you are sitting at the same height and in chairs of similar construction, that the room is comfortably warm and the lighting appropriate. If you have a drink, you both use similar cups.

These basics are the ideal, even the theoretical. We all know that much helping and counselling takes place during bed-bathing and tub-bathing, in linen cupboards, on the doorstep or in noisy dining rooms. But given the chance, often with a minimum of effort, these conditions can be improved. When you are sensitive to the needs of others, they may not even notice that you are helping them in this way.

When you have a chance, notice the effect created when you sit and swivel in your comfortable office armchair, while your client sits in a moulded fibreglass chair, or when your patient is lying down in bed and you sit on the edge. If there is a table between you, clutching the shoulders of someone bursting into tears becomes quite a performance.

Most of all, though, what matters is the quality of your presence. It matters that *you are there*. You are with that person, not with the client you have just left, your evening guests, or what you are about to tell the boss. When you can be with each of these in their own time you will be more effective there and then, and also save yourself a good deal of mental energy.

It is clear that this quality of presence is not always possible to the same degree. It depends on your disposition and on the relationship between two people. But it is also true that part of wanting to help is making every effort to get the conditions right. This may sometimes mean giving yourself a push and wanting to be there, even if this is demanding.

Egan (1994, p. 91) has described the helper's physical attending with the acronym SOLER:

Squarely: Face the client **S**quarely. This can be meant both physically (sitting opposite) and metaphorically (conveying the message 'I am with you').

Open: Adopt an **O**pen posture. Crossed arms and legs can be signs of closing off. Your posture should convey 'I am open to you'.

Lean: It is possible to **L**ean towards the other. Leaning towards the other person can be seen as 'I am interested in you'.

Eye: Maintain **E**ye contact. This is a comfortable contact, not a staring. It is a way of saying 'I am with you; I want to hear what you have to say'.

Relaxed: Try to be **R**elaxed. Nervousness and fidgeting are easily transmitted. This can make an unsure client even more uncomfortable. When you are relaxed, the client can also relax.

None of this is a rule, rather a reminder of aspects of helping which, when you are yourself, you do anyway.

Being non-judgemental

'The highest expression of empathy is accepting and (being) non-judgemental' (Rogers, 1980). Rogers goes on to tell the story of a psychologist who was researching people's visual and perceptual history, including difficulties with seeing and reading. He simply listened to the subjects with interest and so gathered his data. To his surprise a number of them came back to thank him for his help. In his opinion he had given them no help at all. It made him 'recognize that interested non-evaluative listening is a potent therapeutic force'.

You would not survive in life without making judgements. As a nurse you have to make many judgements every day. There is a great difference, though, between judging the speed of an oncoming car when you want to cross the road, and making a judgement about a person. This judgement is probably overlaid with prejudices and stereotypes, fears and values. It is these things that have to be laid aside if a relationship is to be built.

The next time you admit a new patient, be aware of how many judgements you will have formed before you have been with this patient for five minutes. The name, the age, the diagnosis, the handshake, the patient's clothes: these are all ways in which a person is 'revealed'. But these things do not yet make a person.

When you are with a patient or client, you enter that person's world. That may be a very different world from your own. In a sense it is true that feelings of love and hate are the same the world over, but how they are expressed are not. When people are ill, their basic patterns and instincts tend to become more important to them and even become exaggerated. Different customs concerning food and hygiene are now widely acknowledged, but some religious and spiritual practices may not yet be so widely understood.

Perry (1988) makes the point that a helping intervention may be interpreted as 'Babylon' by a Rastafarian, and thus as evidence of the oppression of his or her people. An Asian person may not want to take part in any treatment, including counselling, outside a setting where the whole family is involved; this may apply particularly to women. In that setting, concepts of 'self-determination' and 'self-responsibility' are irrelevant because the culture does not value personal autonomy.

A patient may say that he or she can be washed only at a time when the evil spirits are not around; another converses with the spirits. When the culture and language of a particular patient are not our own, we can be quick to dismiss unfamiliar practices and to impose our own routines and standards.

If you can set aside the patient's name, accent, colour of hair and diagnosis. . .

If you can set aside his need for three sugars in his coffee, his dislike of baths or his rituals when dressing. . .

If you can set aside her use of your least favourite perfume, her constant late arrival, her silly nickname for her husband. . .

If you can hear what he says as being *his* story and his truth. . .

If you can believe what she says, despite what you think. . .

If you can show respect without thinking of how this affects you. . .

If you can do all this, then you are meeting a *person*, not a uniform, a preconceived idea, or a diagnosis.

This patient declared one morning that she needed to be moved to the single room so that she could die in peace. She was ill, but she was not considered to be on the verge of death. Something in her voice took me aback. I could not argue with her. I had a single room available, and I moved her, somehow waiting to be proved wrong. She telephoned all her relatives, one after the other, to come to her bedside. She asked her nephew to help her make a will. She asked him to close her bank account and to have the cash in £5 notes. She wanted to give a present to all who came into her room: doctors, cleaners, nurses, friends, everyone got £5. When all this was done, she simply laid down and died.

You will probably have your own story about the importance of being non-judgemental. If not, think of your patients, and be aware, when you were last judgemental and how much you could help them; and when you were non-judgemental, and the help you were able to give then.

Body language

The non-verbal communication of both people in any interaction is important.

Paying attention to the client's body language can tell you a great deal of what may be going on. Posture, facial expression, breathing, eye contact, nervousness or listlessness – all point to the overall picture presented. Most nurses are very good at observation; you can make use of these aspects for your helping. The five senses are excellent detectives and pointers to the overall picture.

The sense of *sight* can be used very effectively and you can feed this back to a patient.

When you said that you uncrossed your arms. Is it a relief to have said it?
A frown came across your forehead just then – is this something which is troubling you?
Your face brightened up as you said that.
You were looking away then, almost as if you did not want to face this.
That was a deep sigh – what happened there?

The sense of *hearing* is in the listening. You listen not only to the words, but also to the tone of the words, their speed, and how quietly they are spoken. Does the client have a dry mouth? Does speech come easily? Does your client use plain speech or metaphors? Paying attention to what is said and how it is said can give you insights that are useful to you, and that clients give away, probably without being aware of it. Making them aware of this might be a useful tool in helping.

You can also make use of *smell*. You can gain a lot of information from the way both men and women use smells and scents to enhance their image, and which part of that image they enhance or neglect. Clients who are depressed are less likely to use scent and dress well. A counselling relationship, however, may be a turning point, and if you notice a change in appearance, you can comment on it and perhaps a person with a low self-esteem can feel encouraged.

The request 'come and smell my lovely roses' may be an opening for a patient in need of attention. Such an invitation should never be underestimated.

You may not often be called upon to use the sense of *taste*, but you could be in situations when patients and clients offer you sweets, a cup of tea, or some other titbit to eat. This can be an important token of sharing.

Touch, the last sense, plays a considerable part in helping. When you get nearer to people emotionally, you also get nearer physically. Nurses have close physical contact with many people, but this may not be emotional contact. On the whole, neither is it a reciprocal contact: nurses touch patients, but by and large patients do not touch nurses.

Some people who are disturbed and frightened want very close contact; others want to be left alone. When you can read the body language of such people you will probably help in the most appropriate way.

It is perhaps the sense of touch that is the most difficult and also the most pertinent of the senses in helping. Without words you can convey deep caring with an arm around a shoulder. Or you can cradle a person like a child while he or she cries and lets go of tension and pent-up emotions. At such moments you overstep the norms of touching, and barriers of 'right' conduct are forgotten. When you help someone, you do so essentially as another human being, and this is nowhere more clearly demonstrated than in the act of touching and being touched. The language of the body is used not only to reveal aspects of the client's life to you, but you also use it to convey to the client that you are 'with' and 'for' that person.

Your non-verbal communication is as important to patients or clients as theirs is to you. Reading personal signals comes naturally to most people. It is often easier to read the other person's signal than to be aware of the signals we ourselves give. Have you ever watched yourself in a mirror while talking with someone on the telephone? It might be an interesting exercise to do this occasionally. The mere fact that you are watching yourself distracts you from the conversation, and the other person cannot even see this. When the other can actually watch you, it becomes clear how often we are not 'all there'.

Giving space

With understanding and empathy you move into the other's world. This is both a physical and an emotional world.

Nurses know well enough the privileged position they have in the physical territory of patients. They wash people, clean their teeth for them, give them enemas, deliver their babies, change their colostomy bags. Much of this is done to people who are almost, or completely, naked. They are going much closer than even a close family member might go in physical contact. It should not be astonishing, then, that such people also let you into their intimate personal space, or, alternatively, that they resent this and drive you out.

The emotional territory of feelings, experiences and meaning can be compared with a moor, or a wood. There is growth at different levels. There are also unnoticed stones, holes, roots, perhaps caves and ravines. These things need to be experienced and noticed if you both want to journey through this landscape. This is done by the client telling you a story. But the telling of it has to be encouraged.

By patiently listening to the distraught man, by being present for him, we give him space to think and to feel. Perhaps, instead of speaking of space and time, it would be truer to say that the patient man gives the other room to live; he enlarges the other's living room. (Mayeroff, 1971, p. 12)

People need to roam about in their thoughts, go down memory lane and build castles in the air; they need permission to talk and explore the inner country. They may need little more than the occasional word of encouragement; or they may need you as a companion in this exploration.

By being respectful of the other person's physical and emotional space, you give them something vital. You give them, or help them to give themselves, their own selves. You also give them an assurance that they matter.

How much space do you need personally? The awareness you have of your own needs will guide you to help others, although their needs may vary greatly from yours.

Timing and pacing   The time you have available for help will necessarily influence the process of helping itself. When there is pressure, you can do as much work in ten minutes as in one hour and ten minutes. Helping a person with a speech impairment will always take longer than helping someone who can talk normally.

Some clients are themselves quick people; others are slow. Some helpers are more energetic than others. A really deep-seated, painful problem cannot be exposed or explained quickly. On the other hand, some problems are very pressing. Will a patient accept a certain treatment? If not, what are the reasons and available resources for coping otherwise? The parents of a disabled baby may have to decide within hours or days what they think is the best course of action in a given set of circumstances. Other patients may not have to make a decision for some time.

It may be appropriate not only to push patients and clients in a helping situation, but also to slow them down. A quick decision may be a panic decision, and helpers may have to be firm and look at certain unclear or reluctant areas quite decisively.

Some people need far more time with one aspect than with another. It may be unrealistic to think that because yesterday some patients or relatives needed twenty minutes of time, today they will need the same amount of time for a new aspect that may have arisen.

When you are 'with' the person, attending to your client fully, you will be aware of his or her time needs. To have some boundaries can be helpful but boundaries are valid only when they can also be broken.

How does your own pressure of time influence your helping? What messages does this give to clients? It is a truism that half the world has too little time and the other half too much. Fitting these two opposites together in helping is often like juggling. It is perhaps also important to consider whose time is more valuable and what decisions are made around this topic. In a climate of scarce resources, such messages may have far-reaching consequences.

Staying open   By staying open is meant accepting, giving permission to talk, and listening. It is another way of saying 'I am here for you'. It means that, as a helper, you go where the client wants to go. You follow your client's agenda, not yours, although as part of the counselling process you may bring clients to face issues which they may not have intended or even known about.

Patient: I believe there is something better than this at the end of it all, but I don't want to go yet. (Patient suppresses a tear.)
Nurse: It sounds and looks as though you are ready for a good cry.
Patient: That's it, you're right.
Nurse: If you want to cry that's alright by me.
Patient: A bit. But it doesn't do any harm. (Patient cries, then laughs, and cries again.)

By staying open to what is happening, you are not judging a person. You are open and ready to go with the client. Only by staying open will you be able to offer a person the safety to go on talking, or to stop and cry – or laugh. So often, patients come to the brink of talking about something important, delicate or painful, and then stop. 'I mustn't worry you. You might think me morbid.' To say something like, 'You are not worrying me. Tell me about it' will give the necessary permission. It may sound a little 'professional', but depending on the tone of voice and all the other factors of relating, such a moment may be the turning point for a person in emotional distress.

In a way, the skill of staying open sums up all the skills of attending. None of these skills is easy, because they demand that you are all 'there'. By staying open you risk being hurt, becoming involved, getting tired, being exploited and used. But it is only by staying open that you can come close to another person and see change happen. The deep satisfaction in helping is that you can often see such changes and realize that, without your openness and your own vulnerability, this might not have come about, at least not in the same way. The following story shows how important these points are:

She talked and talked and talked. After about 45 minutes she looked at her watch and reached for her shopping bag.
'Well, Doctor, I really must be going, but thank you once again for all the advice – I don't know what I'd do without it.'
For three-quarters of an hour I'd listened to the good lady without saying a single word – *except 'good morning' of course. What is more, it had been just the same each time we'd met over the preceding three months.* (Martin, 1977)

Listening

I listen, hopefully in such a way that the person of my concern will hear, from deep within, the decisions which he or she has to make and act upon. (Kirkpatrick, 1985)

Listening is the beginning, middle and end of helping. The first of the Four Questions 'What is happening?' is the question of and for listening.

Listening is something active. You are not only sitting and letting your ears do the work: you respond and interact with the person with you. You listen with the whole of yourself to the whole of the other person. A client once said to me, 'Thank you for having such big ears'. She clearly did not mean only the ears at the side of my head.

Listening is active in that it hears what is spoken and also not spoken but implied. 'Can't you do something more for this pain?' may in reality be 'You are not taking my pain seriously and I am angry with you for this'. The implication is the anger. Written on paper it may sound flat, but combined with the patient's tone of voice and the look in his or her eyes it is clear what is meant.

What is this person trying to communicate? What is he saying about his feelings? What is she saying with her behaviour? Why is she saying it now and what does it mean?

To *hear* another person is perhaps the biggest gift we can ever give. When you hear someone, you accept him or her unconditionally, without any judgement. When you hear individuals, you give them the means to hear themselves. When you listen in such a way that your clients can hear themselves, then they are able to become themselves and grow.

Listening is active in that it listens *for* something. It listens for the person, for all that she or he expresses. It listens in particular for the feelings expressed or hidden. It listens for the meaning that all this may have for the person. It listens finally for a goal to emerge, and for ways in which the person can or could change.

The essence of empathy is that you hear the other and communicate this back so that you both know that understanding has taken place.

Patient: And if anything happens to him, well, Lord knows what will happen to me. Shoved in a home for geriatrics I suppose. But I mustn't look on that side of things.

Nurse: But you do look on that side. I heard you say things about being useless several times.

Patient: Well, this is it. I do feel useless, and I have never been useless in my life, but, the only thing is, if I can't be useful because I am immobile, then perhaps I can be useful in other ways. There is a nurse over there who has got marital problems, and she was showering me the other day and I got talking to her, and she said I helped. And I thought, well, if I can help people that way it won't be so bad, will it? I shan't be completely useless.

When you listen to the other person you filter through you what is said. You let the words drip *through* you like water; you don't divert the water into your channel.

Patient:	Sister, I know I shouldn't be saying this, but I just can't get on with Nurse N. Can't you find another nurse to look after me?
Nurse:	You don't get on with N?
Patient:	She is rude to me.
Nurse:	Can you be more specific?
Patient:	She always calls me 'little Doris'. I told her I am not 'little'.
Nurse:	She diminishes you.
Patient:	Yes, she makes me feel a child. She treats me as if I were a nitwit.
Nurse:	You are saying that with pain in your voice.
Patient:	(bursts into tears) I've been trying so hard all my life to do the right thing. Somehow, she has managed to get where it hurts most.
Nurse:	What does doing the right thing mean for you?
Patient:	Do you really want to listen to a long story?
Nurse:	Sounds like you need to tell it – go on please.

This edited and shortened conversation (which did not finish where the extract ends) shows several of the points made in this chapter:

The full acceptance of the client without judging her or diverting from her subject.
The nurse gave her the space and time she needed. The many 'um's and 'ah's and pauses used would make this point more clearly.
She gave the patient permission to talk.
She encouraged her.
She helped her to get to her own strong point: 'doing the right thing'.
With that she was into the area of meaning for and in her life.

Listening is hearing a great deal, and often not saying much. (A posture can sometimes say just as much.)

Nature gave man two ears but only one tongue, which is a gentle hint, that he should listen more than he talks. (Davis, 1972)

Encouraging

Anything unexpected, particularly illness and loss, usually leads to some loss of confidence.

I was managing alright, now I just can't.
I thought I was doing so well, until this happened.
I can't see my way through this at all.
I feel such a fool not being able to make up my mind.

Such loss of confidence may be temporary, or it may be the beginning of a downward slide into incompetence. One way of compensating is by becoming aggressive. Another is to abandon oneself to the 'sick' role, or to revert to childlike behaviour. Many people give an impression of self-assurance but when it comes to the crunch they are as helpless as those far less confident.

A blocked and paralysed person cannot move forward and change anything. A person who has no self-trust cannot imagine that life could be different.

The first step in any kind of helping is usually an awareness exercise. For whatever reason, someone who needs help is like a china doll. It was a beautiful doll, but something or someone smashed it up. It is lying in pieces on the floor. Parts of it are perfectly recognizable. But it cannot put itself together again on its own.

A glued-together doll will always be fragile and probably ugly. But a shattered person who is helped to come together again is much stronger for the experience. Nevertheless, some people do remain broken, scarred and in pieces. For whatever reason, they have chosen that path. People can be 'mended'; that is, they can have operations to correct diseased parts, and they can have medications to put some other aspect of the body right again. But they remain 'dolls'. They are not fully alive because the purpose of being ill does not exist any more. Such people can be approached only with compassion, not with a zeal to change them. Real empathy accepts a person, and in that very acceptance may lie the seed for change.

The person who is able and willing to allow you to help him or her to gather the pieces together has already taken a vital first step. As a helper it is important (to continue with the metaphor) to point out and look at the pieces that are still intact, or the large bits that are clearly visible. Your help will enable them to see these pieces too. Very often a vital early step in helping is to encourage clients to discover the parts or pieces that are still together and strong. This gives them the confidence to go on and also to search for other such parts or areas of their lives which work well.

The skill of encouraging is firmly based in the helper attitudes of being hopeful and supportive. It is particularly relevant when considering that helping does not mean filling an empty vessel with wisdom, but building on the client's own strengths and calling forth the client's own resources. It also means giving the message 'I believe in you; I trust you'. Moments of discouragement will always be with us, but the important thing is that this is not all there is. There is more to a person than the present obvious difficulty. The person is not all failure.

Encouragement is much more, therefore, than a slap on the back. It is a fundamental skill of helping without which most of us would be poor and helpless. Before any helping or actual counselling, and therefore changing, can be done, what is already there has to be seen and strengthened. Not only does what a client sees and tells you need to be encouraged: the whole person needs to be encouraged.

As with so much on the subject of helping, the skills described here are nothing more than basic human interacting. We will have learnt that in the nursery. If you see it as professional work, you are in danger of becoming aloof and distanced. But if you are not professional you are in danger of being flippant. How do you keep the balance? That is a question only you can answer for yourself. But the answer you give is an important element in the way you help others.

CHAPTER EIGHT

Counselling skills: assessing

....

Assessing

Nurses are well acquainted with the term assessment from the nursing process. The first step in this process is to assess the situation and base the care that the client needs on this assessment. In a similar way, this is what is happening at the beginning of a helping relationship.

I use the term 'helping relationship' in its widest sense. In particular, this means also any interaction where counselling skills are used but which is not called counselling, and also for those situations that are clearly counselling relationships. If it is an interaction of a few minutes or a few meetings, at the beginning there is necessarily some assessment going on.

The assessment I mean here is about establishing what the problem is and what the client needs from the helper and the helper needs from the client. The relationship between the two people can then be formed, for however short or long a time this may be.

The helper is the person addressed and sought as someone with knowledge or skills, or both, to help the client. The client says in effect, 'I don't know, please help me'. Admitting this helplessness may be quite difficult and even embarrassing for some clients. The helper may also be put in a situation of presumed knowledge or skill which can be unrealistic.

Assuming that the helper can and wants to help presupposes that she or he has the skills necessary. The helper then uses those skills to help the other person to tell the story. As the story unfolds the helper responds by pointing out strengths and weaknesses in self-help skills which the client has. The assessing is therefore not like the nursing process where a great many details are asked, many of which may be irrelevant and those that might be relevant are often not asked for and thus not supplied.

Assessing is not just a question and answer session. It is a situation where two human beings meet as people. Their sharing enhances them. The helper initially shares the application of some specific skills; the client shares information that will enhance the helping. The focus is on the client, but the helper who is 'used' correctly also gains.

Since this helping is based on emotional material rather than simply factual information, there is a possibility that the information given is distorted, unclear and only partly revealed. The helper's job is not to get every last detail out of a client before giving help; the helper's job is to facilitate the telling of the story in as relevant a way as possible. This involves much exploring for the client.

Exploring

If the journey is as important as arriving at the destination, then exploring the landscape over which the road goes is inevitably included in this picture. With the exploration goes discovery. Frankl (1962, p. 101) believes that meaning is only ever *discovered*, not created, by a person. To discover that meaning, a considerable amount of exploring has to be done.

Exploring the world of a person can be like exploring uncharted land. The client may know some important places and stopping points in this world, but not how she or he gets to them. The helper may have a compass, but the client has to lead the helper to the places the compass points to. The compass points steadily in the direction of the client's inner strength, potential and fulfilment.

This analogy makes it clear that the two people in a helping relationship are on this journey together. For the client it is the life journey and the helper is there as companion: the person 'with bread', that is, someone who is willing to share what he or she has.

The exploring to be done in helping concerns both factual events and inner feelings and meanings. Since most problems that need help concern a relationship, the facts are the visible elements, but the inner feelings constitute the actual problem. The relationship with another person often only mirrors the relationship to and with ourselves. It is probably true to say that most problems arise out of the relationship we have with ourselves. Helping a client, therefore, almost always means leading the client from the outside to the inside of the story; helping the client to 'personalise the experience' (Carkhuff); looking for 'leverage' (Egan); and asking 'What is the meaning of it?' Some permission has to be given in order that exploring can start. But eventually the movement has to be to the outside again by some action that changes the client's thinking and behaving: 'How are you going to do it?'

Allowing

Perhaps the most obvious element in helping is that helping is allowed to happen. Without necessarily saying so, the helper gives the client permission to talk. When this permission is not given, no connection can be made and no helping takes place. It is possible that helpers take it for granted that they have given permission and it is also possible that clients dare not take the permission. The process has to begin somewhere, however that permission to tell the story is given.

Fabun (1968, in Navone 1977, p. 27) believes that no experience ever begins. There was always something that went before. The only thing that begins is the person's awareness of something going on. In a sense, therefore, every story always begins with 'and'. This can be infuriating for people who like things neatly wrapped up, but it can be liberating for those who know that they can never really reach an end, only a new beginning. Perhaps every story should therefore also end with 'and'.

This little word 'and' is also the word of relationships: 'You and me'; 'I and Thou'. It is the word that most of us need to learn to say more sincerely.

Allowing individuals to tell their story is not only good and helpful for them: by doing so you allow yourself to be open to each person whose story you hear. In this way you affirm both yourself and the other. On this affirmation the desire to change can be built.

The story-telling is the first stage of the present scenario (Egan); the responding to clients (Carkhuff); and the Developing of the relationship (Nelson-Jones). It is the very tip of the question 'What is happening?' Very often the client does not know what the problem actually is, or is not sufficiently in touch with it. For the problem to be described and defined, the story may have to be described in considerable detail; or it may have to be taken back further and further – more and more 'ands' have to be added. This may mean going down memory lanes, up garden paths, through long, dark corridors, opening doors here and there, looking around corners and turning over every stone. No wonder our language is full of such images!

In that telling, things are not only clarified but also healed. Most bereaved persons have to tell the story of the death or loss many times over. Each telling of the story allows some details to be changed, emerge, or be dropped, and in that change it becomes more part of the person. 'The outer journey is the plot; the inner journey is the meaning' (Navone, 1977, p. 69).

Some people have no particular sense of journey. They see life as a succession of events which happen to them. In being allowed to tell the story of these events, shapes may begin to emerge, patterns can be recognized, and links made between happenings that never seemed to be related. In this way some meaning which may have been hidden for years may begin to emerge. Such meanings are often the strong points in a person's life which help him or her to keep going, sometimes against all odds. They are what makes a person 'tick'.

The skills that the helper needs are those of giving permission to talk, encouraging the continuation of the story-telling, being unafraid of what might emerge, and listening for that which matters and has meaning in the person's life.

The client too has to be unafraid: unafraid of actually telling the story. Some people feel that their story is so awful that they dare not repeat it. If they want to be helped then they have to say what they need help with.

Peter was an 18-year-old with suspected cancer of the testes. He asked his nurse to tell him what the prognosis was for this kind of cancer.

Nurse: I could give you facts and figures. Is that what you want?
Peter: Not only.
Nurse: How else can I help you?
Peter: Well, I wondered ... You see, I am ... Oh, I can't really tell you ....
Nurse: It's all right, tell me what you can. I'll do the same.

The nurse was not quite sure why Peter had asked that particular question as she knew that he was well informed about tests and treatments, so her question was directed to the *person*, not just the problem. To allow him to say a bit more, she was therefore deliberately open at the beginning. By saying later that she, too, will tell Peter as much as she can, she made a kind of 'pact' with him to collaborate, and that may have given Peter the security to be as open as possible.

If the nurse had simply concentrated on the 'problem' presented, i.e. the prognosis, she might have said something like:

Nurse: That depends on many things and it's too early to be sure at this moment.

Peter would probably never have said anything more.

Allowing means allowing 'things' to happen and events to develop. In this case the nurse got quite a story.

Seeking information

Help given can be based only on the information available. The helper's skill at the beginning of an interaction is to help clients to tell their story. They in turn are helped by hearing themselves recount what happened or how things are.

This topic is mentioned here as a helper skill, which it clearly is in the way the information is sought. But it must be pointed out that the information looked for is largely used by the helper to understand the client and the situation. But the client, in being encouraged to tell the story, also learns from the way the story is told, or what is not told.

The personality plays a large part in how and what information is sought and given. Some extroverted people will always give information freely while some introverted people may respond only to prompts. On the other hand, introverted people may also talk more freely about feelings and their inner world and neglect making connections with tangible events. But asking extroverted people to relate some event to an inner meaning may sound ridiculous to them. When this happens, helpers can relate this to the person and the wider picture which thus emerges, possibly giving clues to what might be blind spots and blockages to change.

It is impossible to give isolated examples of the skills detailed in this chapter without showing other skills at the same time, but in particular this always refers also to empathy. An example of seeking information may therefore also be clarifying or summarizing, and it is certainly empathic.

Patient: I could really do with having my daughter here now.
Nurse: Does she live far away?
Patient: No, not really, but. . .
Nurse: But. . .
Patient: Well, we just don't get on with each other.
Nurse: Say a bit more about that.

To help this client, the nurse needed to have more information about the daughter first of all, and then about the relationship the client has with his daughter. It may be quite feasible that the patient gave his daughter's name and address as next of kin when the nursing assessment was made, but there might have been nothing to indicate then that they did not get on with each other. It may not have been an issue then; clearly it is now.

The information which a helper is looking for should relate to the story and the actual problem. There is no merit in having much information which is not relevant. Prompting may be useful in getting the right information, but prying is not therapeutic. (Stewart, 1992, p. 131)

When seeking information, the most obvious tool to use is questioning. But questions are not always appropriate, as they can let the client do less work and rely only on your questions. Much information can be sought without asking questions, but giving small prompts: 'Tell me more'; 'Go on'; 'I am not sure whether I quite understood that'. When questions are used, it matters therefore *how* they are used.

Questioning

You may have to ask for further information when a client's story is unclear. What seems clear to the client may not be so clear to anybody else. The types of questions you ask, and how you ask them, will be crucial for the information you get.

A look at questions in general is therefore called for.

According to Tomlinson (1983) the functions of questions are:

1. Gathering information.
2. Encouraging conversation.
3. Identifying problems and difficulties.
4. Focusing attention on specific issues or topics.
5. Expressing interest in others.
6. Discovering attitudes and opinions of others.

The skill of questioning is in the way questions and behaviour, tone and attitude, blend. In helping and counselling, questions are used to get to a goal. For this reason open and closed questions are useful, but open questions concentrate on the client whereas closed ones display more often the helper's agenda.

Open questions leave respondents free to answer as they wish. They are broad in nature, but are more time-consuming, and answers may contain irrelevant but valuable and unexpected information.

The first of the Four Questions, 'What is happening?', is a completely open question. It is a free invitation to clients to tell their story. According to Stewart (1992, p. 188), open questions beginning with 'could' 'tend to be the most open and help clients generate their own unique answers':

Could you tell me a bit more about this?

Questions beginning with 'what' 'tend to bring out the specific facts of a problem':

What is happening?
What is the meaning of it?
What is your goal?
What do you make of this?

'How' questions 'often lead toward discussion'. When the word 'feel' is included the client is usually more ready to talk about feelings:

How do you feel about your daughter?
How are you going to do it?

Stewart (1992, p. 188) says that 'why' questions 'tend to lead clients to talk about their past or present reasoning around an event or situation'. 'Why' questions are normally closed questions. While they have their place in helping and counselling, clearly they should be used with caution because they may give the impression of an interrogation.

Other types of questions can be leading, process and rhetorical. Perhaps the type of question most to avoid is a multiple one, when several questions are asked without giving the client a chance to answer each: 'Have you lived there long? Do you like it? I mean, what are the neighbours like?' Usually only the last question gets answered.

It is quite possible that what a client says may bring several further questions or points to mind. Helpers who handle questions well may then say something like:

This points to three things that seem important: you feel pretty awful at the moment and I would like to know more about that; you wish there were someone to help you sort out this insurance business; and I wonder whether there might not also be a problem with your stomach.

This example shows the skills of summarizing, clarifying and reflecting. It also shows that questions can be asked in a non-confrontative way. If there are several questions presenting themselves, putting the matter in such a detailed fashion gives the client the choice to respond to what seems most important or most appropriate.

Experiencing feelings

As the counselling type of helping is directed towards problem management (rather than problem solving), it is clear that much of the attention has to be on the feelings involved. Some people have great difficulty in separating feelings and thinking. If you ask them, 'How do feel about this?', they will answer, 'I think that it is wrong'.

Accessing feelings is quite foreign to many people. They believe that feelings are dangerous, that they are 'women's problems' or that they never feel anything or indeed need to feel anything at all. Despite today's greater emphasis on feelings for both men and women, the actual understanding of feelings, what they do to us and how we handle them, has not really changed. In times of crisis most of us act out of well-established patterns.

One man, who was in hospital for a short spell during a long-term illness, learnt that his wife had left him for his next-door neighbour. When asked how he felt, he repeatedly replied, 'I don't feel anything. She walked out'.

Such statements need to be heard and acknowledged because they say much about the person and where this person is 'at' at this moment. This patient *may* not have been feeling anything because he was shocked and numbed, and this led him to deny having any responsibility in his wife's decision to leave.

Other people are just the opposite. They believe themselves to be ruled by their heart rather than their head. Yet others might identify with the gut and function from there. Any of these basic locations of drives is normal; they become problematic only when people feel or think that they cannot control or change this.

Clearly, all people have feelings, but we are not all the same in the way we experience them or deal with them. Helping clients to get in touch with their feelings is therefore often an important task early in helping. Those who hide their feelings may need to recognize that feelings play a large role in their lives, and those who are or feel themselves to be ruled by their feelings may need to see them in perspective.

One way of helping patients and clients to centre around their experiences is to ask them to make 'I statements'. This is particularly indicated for people who say 'you' or 'one' about themselves.

You go through with this treatment and at the end you feel worse than ever.
Can you say this as 'I'?
I had this treatment and at the end I felt worse than before.

Using 'you' or 'one' can be a technique used by clients to distance themselves from the real experience, and this can lead to an impossibility of dealing with problems effectively. Asking clients to say 'I' is a form of challenge. It is also an important way of showing that you mean business, that is, you are helping, not just sympathizing.

Another way of getting in touch with feelings is by asking patients and clients where in the body they locate particular feelings. If this is not helpful, it may be useful to ask them where in the body they now experience tension. This may point to the kind of feelings that may be associated with such tensions.

Since we are what we feel, it may be true to say that we are tense when we experience tension somewhere in the body. Someone who is not feeling happy *is* not happy. It is not just the mood that is not happy; the whole body is not happy.

Sometimes people simply find it impossible to talk about their feelings. Fraser (1990) has shown that by encouraging her pregnant clients to write down their feelings as letters or stories she was able to help them significantly by reading the lines, and between them, to discover what mattered most. This is a possibility that could be used in any setting.

Feelings are as varied as life itself. There are the generally recogniz-able feelings of fear, anger, sadness, despair, joy, embarrassment, love, frustration, and so on. But there are many other feelings which have no particular name, and of which everybody is differently aware. There are levels or degrees of feelings. Being pleased is weaker than being excited, though it is still a feeling of happiness. (Tschudin, 1994, p. 42)

Helping clients and patients to own their feelings and take responsibility for them is often the central aspect of helping. Being in charge of our feelings, rather than feelings being in charge of us, or denying feelings, means that there is holistic living. At this point in the helping relationship the emphasis is on recognizing and experiencing feelings.

It may therefore be necessary to ask questions relating to feeling both frequently and in different ways:

What are you feeling about that?
How do you feel now?
What does that bring up in the way of feelings?
Have you always felt like that?
Do you have other feelings besides this one?

When do you feel like this particularly?

The following discussion with a patient touches on several feelings. Notice how they were dealt with.

Patient: Do you think that death is as taboo a subject now as sex was in Victorian times?

Nurse: Probably, yes.

Patient: I have to make a confession: I have never seen a dead body, not even my father when he died. I rationalize it; I was afraid.

Nurse: How do you feel about death now?

Patient: I'm afraid of pain. If I have to die...

Nurse: You are afraid of pain?

Patient: More than death, actually. The thought of pain – I'd do anything to be rid of it.

Nurse: What sort of pain are you afraid of?

Patient: Nagging pain.

Nurse: Nagging pain?

Patient: Nag, nag, nag, all day, without relief.

Nurse: Like the boss you told me about yesterday who nags you.

Patient: Funny – yes, I hadn't made the connection.

Acknowledging and staying with the feelings can open all sorts of doors. Many people are rightly afraid that facing their feelings may lead them into the dark recesses of their lives where they can get lost. This is a realistic enough fear and one that might need help from a qualified counsellor or psychiatrist. Most helping situations do not go to such depths, but the basic helper attitudes of hopefulness and support are there precisely for such possibilities.

As the helper you go with your clients into the darkness or the unknown place. As the companion on the road you have made a commitment for the duration of the interaction or relationship and you may need to assure your clients of this. When they know and realize that you are there, they may begin to experience their feelings and take responsibility for them.

Clarifying

The goal of helping is to give clients an opportunity to work at living and functioning in a more satisfying and resourceful way, and one which eventually leads to self-responsibility and self-therapy by clients. Many of the helping situations that we meet start out with the client being very unclear: 'I don't know what's the matter with me, but I'm not feeling very well today'. The immediate goal is therefore to clarify what is going on. Unless the client is clear what the problem is, decisions as to what to do about it cannot be made.

The skill of clarifying is to help the client see a situation more clearly, understand a problem more precisely, or simply get more insight in a skilled way. Thus clarifying is often a basic tool for helping. It clarifies something for the client, but in the process the helper also gains in that his or her task is easier after a clear start.

The first response to an unclear statement is therefore often one of clarification.

In what way are you not feeling well?
Can you tell me what it is you *are* feeling?

After some initial unfolding of the story and therefore the problem, the important issues can then be elucidated. Any problem situation is made up of experiences, behaviours and feelings, and active listening will help to clarify these. Helping becomes useful only when there are specific things to concentrate on. The aim is to work towards a goal.

One of the ways in which counselling is diminished is by making assumptions. Before you make a decision in your own mind that your client is this or that sort of person, or that you know exactly what the problem is, check it out.

Patient: I have never been sure that my mother loved me.
Nurse: a) How did your mother treat you?
    b) What makes you unsure of her love?
    c) What sort of a relationship did you have with your mother?
    d) Is this a statement or are you trying to understand something here?

Nelson-Jones' (1993, p. 23) distinction between 'self-talk' and 'public talk' is useful here. The 'self-talk' may here include thoughts like:

How I know that problem!
Is it better to share something of my own problem or not?
This could be his reason for not functioning well now.
Do I need to know more about this problem?
How can I best help this person?

Such thinking is essential as it helps you sort the useful from the useless. It also means that, for instance, if a client mentions something that is close to your own emotions, you can decide what to do. The statement, 'I have never been sure that my mother loved me' may be true for many people, and hearing it said by a client may now bring up strong feelings in you as a helper. Thinking skills may then be essential in deciding: 'I must share a similar position with this client as it might help him'; or 'I must share a similar position with this client as it will help me to deal with my strong feelings'; 'I don't need to say anything about my own emotions at the moment'; 'Being aware of my own emotions at the moment is enough to cope with this situation'. From such thinking will come an accurate use of helper skills, that is, the skills used may be reflecting, focusing, self-sharing or clarifying.

The various ways of clarifying will help the client to spell out, perhaps for the first time, what had until then been only an amorphous mass which could not be controlled. By looking at this mass in more detail and more clarity it may become less overwhelming and more manageable.

Some examples of how to clarify are:

Patient:	I'm not very well today.
Nurse:	In what way are you not well?
Patient:	I don't know what's going on with me.
Nurse:	Can you be more specific?
Patient:	I am not in control of myself.
Nurse:	What does it mean for you to be in control of yourself?
Patient:	It will be alright in the end.
Nurse:	What in particular will be alright?
Patient:	Things keep going wrong.
Nurse:	What sort of things keep going wrong?

Paraphrasing

Paraphrasing is an expression that is not much used these days. It is a skill that shares much with clarifying and reflecting. The skill consists of repeating the client's last few words in a slightly different way:

Patient:	I was anxious not to get into that the same trouble again.
Nurse:	You were anxious to avoid a repeat performance.

The main use and purpose of the skill of paraphrasing is in staying with the client's actual words, neither interpreting them nor orienting the process in a direction that might not be the one the client wants or intends. When it is used effectively it demonstrates to the client that the helper has understood the content of the message being communicated. The danger of paraphrasing is that it is used parrot-fashion, that is, always repeating the last few words the client just said. This can become annoying and then serves no particular purpose. As always, a skill is a skill only when used appropriately.

Reflecting

Reflecting is perhaps the most widely known and useful skill of helping.

Reflecting is the active skill of empathy and thus has a subjective element to it. It is not merely the client's words that are reflected back – though it may include these – but there is an attempt to tell clients that you have understood their world. In this way you give 'back' to clients something they might not actually have said, but implied.

Patient: I can't use the time the way I would like to. That's the worst part.

Nurse: It seems as if wasting time is something that is an important issue for you.

Patient: I could do a lot of reading, but I can't read. And I could prepare work, but it just packs in on me. I can't think, and people say to me, it's about time you laid back and thought a while.

Nurse: It sounds as though you are finding your own company quite difficult.

For this patient 'wasting time' was the problem he could talk about, but underneath lay the difficulty of not accepting his illness. This had been picked up by the nurse in previous conversations, but had never been given a name, a 'handle', or a 'lever' (Egan's term) before.

The skill of reflecting concentrates on the feelings and other subjective emotions or states within the statements made by clients. This means that an empathic understanding is there. The skill is then to reflect either a significant word or concept so that the client can move forward into exploring another, and perhaps deeper, aspect of the problem. This is always done with the aim of encouraging awareness, self-responsibility and self-help skills in clients.

When empathy is shown to clients, the focus is the person of the client, not just the problem presented. This is usually characterized by the reflection of feelings: when feelings are addressed, then the person is addressed.

Patient: But I was so desperate to find an answer, and if possible an easy one. I thought, ah well, it's just a little lump in the elbow and they can just remove it and all will be well.

Nurse: You were desperate though.

A psychiatric patient repeatedly said that she *must* change her attitude. She constantly made plans for changing her environment, believing that everything would then be all right. This usually worked for a few days, then her environment was again not conducive to changing her attitudes. She sought help from all who came into contact with her but then usually rejected any help offered. In the example below she was helped to recognize her feelings and work with them by concentrating first on another aspect of her self, which was addressed empathically:

Patient: I really need to get through this. I am on the brink of losing everything and it's just. . .

Nurse: Stop a minute. You just said something important there. You said 'I need to get through this'.

Patient: (slowly) Yes, I must get through this.

Nurse: You said, 'I *need* to get through'.

Patient: Did I?

Nurse: You said 'need'.

Patient: Yes, sure, I must get through it, how else will it work?

Nurse: You *need* to.

Patient: I need to.

Nurse: Is there, I wonder, a difference between needing to and must?

Patient: I hadn't thought about it.

Nurse: Can you see a difference?

Patient: Well, when I say 'need' I am aware of an energy here (pointing to her gut), and when I say 'must', it is more of a head thing.

Nurse: What does the gut energy tell you?

Patient: This is where the *energy* is. The head is not energy. I need to go with the energy, the feeling. That's the real 'me'.

This patient was gradually helped to see that her own *need* was more personal and instinctual, whereas her *must* was an intellectual proposition, picked up from what others around her had said to her.

This interaction shows that sometimes reflecting just one word or concept which matters will bring a person to the necessary insight.

The following is an extract from a discussion with a patient in a rehabilitation unit where he had gone after a spell in another hospital.

Patient: In the other hospital there was a group of us at one stage and we got on incredibly well. But that's different here.

Nurse: Are you saying that you are lonely here?

Patient: Oh no, not lonely. But I do miss talking over the problems from school every day with my wife (they were both teachers). Discussing and working things out together.

Nurse: You are missing something – something you identify with.

Patient: Talking and discussing has always been something I identified with.

Nurse: You have lost something to identify with. Does that point to
            actually having lost your identity?
Patient: You could say that.
Nurse: What does your identity mean to you?

This interaction shows not only the skill of reflecting, but
also clarifying ('are you lonely?'); listening (the words and concepts are heard); the experience of feelings is asked for; 'what
is happening?' is explored; 'what is the meaning of it?' ('what
does your identity mean to you?') is also explored; empathy is
shown in that the whole interaction shows that client and
helper work together; warmth, genuineness and a non-judgemental attitude are also conveyed. When these elements are
present, the problems may begin to be acknowledged and
described, and goals may emerge.

If this is to happen, then the skill of reflecting is not used
only by the helper. The clients too, have to do a good deal of
reflecting: of their situations, their problems, their perceptions,
their attitudes, beliefs and values. Only in this way can helping
be of any use.

Stewart (1992, p. 234) lists some aspects which make
reflecting effective:

1. Observe facial and bodily movements
2. Listen to words and their meanings
3. Tune into your own emotional reactions to what the client
    is communicating
4. Sense the meaning of the communication
5. Take into account the degree of client self-awareness
6. Respond appropriately
7. Use expressive, not stereotyped, language
8. Use vocal and bodily language that agree with each other
9. Check the accuracy of your understanding

This list encompasses many, if not all, the skills described
in more detail in these chapters. It therefore shows what an
important and all-round skill reflecting is.

Guiding to new perspectives

Counsellors can help clients to a new understanding of behaviour and psychological processes and so to new perspectives.
One of the ways of doing this is by interpreting the clients'
world to them. But this skill needs to be used with care. It is
easy to make an interpretation and so give clients the
impression that you know something about them which eludes
them. Many of our blind spots and blocks are due to our own

faulty interpretations of situations, problems and people. Interpreting them in a new way for clients is therefore needed, but the interpretation has to come from within themselves. If you can help your clients to do this by making connections between events and patterns, or between their actions and wider psychological understanding, then this is an effective use of the skill of interpretation. This can often be done initially by giving them information that will be helpful to them in making their own interpetations.

The following conversation took place in a radiotherapy ward:

Patient: I'm slightly disappointed that the treatment isn't going to finish in three weeks but in four weeks, but I think I'm just looking at the need now and accept that.

Nurse: There is a book which points out some steps people who are seriously ill go through. One is anger: why me?

Patient: Oh goodness, yes!

Nurse: One is bargaining: if I am good now, maybe God will be good to me.

Patient: Yes (laughs).

Nurse: One is depression and this is qualified somewhat. But I am using these stages for your situation here.

Patient: Yes, go on.

Nurse: One day you'll be angry, the next day you'll be bargaining, the next you'll be happy.

Patient: Absolutely, I had just that. My weekend consisted more or less of incredible oscillations of that nature. I went through that series, absolutely.

Nurse: Does this help you to accept better what is happening to you?

Patient: It makes all the difference! I can live with myself again and with the disappointment that the treatment takes longer than anticipated.

This kind of interpretation helped the patient to see that his disappointments and reactions to them were quite normal and that he was not 'going mad' because one moment he felt this, and another the opposite. It helped him to see himself, his disease and his treatment in perspective.

The starting point here was actually a text about death and dying (Kübler Ross, 1969), but the nurse noticed a connection between this patient's present position and need for acceptance. The patient was clearly helped by the nurse's knowledge of psychological stages and patterns and by her ability to interpret these to the patient in this particular way.

Interpretation is frequently used in psychotherapy and

analysis, where the therapist interprets repressed or unconscious material such as dreams, visions, fantasies and metaphors, usually within the frame of reference of a particular theory or school. If this is attempted by amateur or would-be helpers, it can be hurtful and possibly damaging:

Your problem is that you never accepted that you couldn't do that job and now everybody is suffering from your bad management.

This statement may be entirely true, but it does not help the person to do anything positive. It may simply show an insecurity or impatience on the part of the helper which the client could interpret in turn as not being the focus of attention and empathy.

An interpretation should be a moving-on statement, on the client's level of understanding. With empathy – being with – it is unlikely that it can go wrong.

Focusing

The assessing skills are broadly there to help clients tell their stories. All this is with the aim in mind that at the end of the interaction clients are in a better or more comfortable place than at the beginning, able to function as independently and resourcefully as possible. Therefore something has to shift. The skill of focusing can help in this.

Focusing can be pictured like a pyramid: there is a wide base of unresolved material and problems. As they are examined and talked about, there is a shaping taking place, narrowing all the time to perhaps one or two goals.

Clients who are 'in a state', or perhaps shocked or disoriented through some loss, are usually not able to think or act clearly and may need help. The skill of focusing is then very useful. Anyone in a severely shocked state is not able to do a great deal of emotional work, therefore the basic skill is to seek a simple way forward or some practical work or action that will help the client to get a grip on the situation. The movement in this skill is to go from the simple to the complex by dealing first with the immediate crisis or problem.

When clients are not necessarily shocked but still unable to handle a particular problem themselves, the skill of focusing is useful in developing the self-helping skills necessary. Egan (1994, p. 220) asks two questions which are quite similar to the Four Questions model: 'What do you want?' and 'What do you have to do to get what you want?' Both these questions help to keep the focus on clients and their needs. Indeed, the skill of focusing may be mainly one of asking relevant questions:

Patient: No matter what I do, I always get it wrong.
Nurse: What had you actually been trying to do?

Patient: I don't know how I can handle this.
Nurse: What are your usual ways of handling difficult situations?

Patient: I am not sure that I can trust myself.
Nurse: Is trusting yourself normally difficult for you?

Patient: It has potential as a way forward.
Nurse: Does this give you some ideas for other possible ways forward?

The skill of focusing is definitely goal-oriented, and this orientation has to start very early on. Telling their story is important for all clients, but simply rambling on is not necessarily helpful – unless that is the purpose of talking. If helping is to be really helpful, there has to be substance to it. Focusing is part of the other skills of assessing, and it overlaps with them in that it is a type of exploring, clarifying, reflecting and summarizing.

Summarizing

Egan (1994, p. 190) says that summarizing provides both focus and challenge. It is partly a 'bridging-skill' between the various stages and is also useful when there might be a point reached where a session or relationship is not advancing, or is stuck. It is not necessarily a good ending for a session as it is not an evaluation.

The technique of making a summary in helping can focus scattered thoughts and feelings. It can also close the conversation on a particular theme, or it can prompt clients to explore a particular theme more thoroughly.

Nurse: If I have understood you rightly, you said that you had had all the tests and they were all negative. Nevertheless, you have a pain which persists. You think this pain is linked with something from the past but you are afraid to look into the past. Is this correct?

A summary can be a mixture of what was said and implied. Summarizing is a 'directing' skill. When clients are directionless, as is quite frequent early on in a helping situation, this skill helps to gather it together. Also, in the early stages there is necessarily a lot of information passed between the two people, and some of it may be confused, or there may be gaps in it which are clear to the client but not necessarily to the helper. Making a summary can then help you from getting lost in either too few or too many details.

The skill of summarizing also has a quality of 'Where do we go from here?' about it. Through no fault of the helper, the client may have become stuck in a thought process or a particular feeling and the conversation seems to be going round in circles. The question 'What is happening?' is applicable then. In this sense it can be seen as a challenge and this will be discussed in Chapter 9 under the skill of immediacy. Making a summary of what has gone on so far may help the larger picture to come into view, by pulling the various topics or strands together. It may then be possible to focus again on what may be happening or may have newly emerged, and this can act like a springboard for further work.

Summarizing helps clients to get a sense of movement. When an insight has been gained or something is seen in a new light, the effect of this is lost if it is not noticed. When these things can be gathered in a few words or sentences, they can be held more easily by clients, thought about, and used in the immediate future, or after the session. It must not be forgotten that the effect of helping and counselling goes on long after the conversation is ended. Indeed, most of the work done may be after the talking has stopped.

CHAPTER NINE

Counselling skills: challenging

Blockages to change

This chapter starts with a short overview of some of the blockages to change which helpers and counsellors encounter.

Sometimes it seems that we are like flies on a window, buzzing around, making a great deal of noise, expending vast amounts of energy, acting as if the window would thereby go away, when only a few inches away a window is open and we could fly through it. The behaviours and attitudes that this picture represents prevent us from moving even a very short distance.

It is important that helpers are sure what they need to challenge. It is the blind spots, the self-defeating patterns of thinking and behaving, the discrepancies and contradictions, and often the unused potential that need to be addressed. It may be outmoded values, old 'baggage' and attitudes that have become irrelevant, but which clients cling to tenaciously, that need to be taken into the real light of day and seen for what they are. As so often, this is far from easy. Berne (1964) chose the title of his book well: *Games People Play*. When the games we play maintain us in illusions, then we may indeed have to be challenged.

The difficulty with these elements is precisely that they are not recognized by clients. Helpers may be alert and spot them very quickly, but clients may take a lot of challenging until they also recognize their existence and relevance. But all of us know how hard it is to be told a truth about ourselves. Therefore challenging has to be done carefully and with empathy.

The blockages to change are the *inconsistencies* in people's lives: inconsistencies between what they say and do; what they think they do and really do; who they imagine themselves to be and who they really are. This last is particularly often evident in people who think they are assertive, whereas in fact they are either manipulative or destructive.

You do as I tell you (but don't do as I do).

Some people adopt *defence mechanisms* to avoid dealing with difficulties. This can show itself in adopting a helpless or hopeless attitude. The position of 'victim' is often met in such people. Patients with serious illnesses may take on an attitude of having no control over the situation, or a negative outcome of a prognosis is experienced as if it had already come about.

There is nothing more that they can do, I might as well opt out now.

Entertaining *negative thoughts* is another feature of blockages to change. Here is an example of two nurses reminiscing about their training days:

A: Isn't it funny how one seems to remember only the demeaning things.
B: That's what *you* remember.
A: But . . .
B: I remember the crises, and they weren't necessarily 'bad'.
A: I never thought of it like that.

Irrational beliefs can be powerful stoppers of change. They distort reality:

I must get through this.
There is a conspiracy going on against me.
I must act in such a way that they will love me.
I cannot let the side down, especially not here.
I cannot be treated in this way.
People who harm me must be blamed and punished.
I must pay now for what I did in the past.
My father taught me never to give in and I cannot let him down.

Such beliefs set up inner rules that lead to irrational consequences. It can at times be very difficult to realize that such rules exist, and even more difficult to let go of them.

Two common ways of blocking change are resistance and avoidance. Most of us will at some stage have said that, when patients begin to resist care or treatment, they are getting better.

As with other defence mechanisms, there is a reason why a person is *resistant* to change. A person may be a 'professional resister', rebelling against any system; or think that needing help is admitting defeat; or feel the need for personal power and express it by resisting someone considered to be more powerful.

I am not going to take this medicine ever.
Yes, but...

Avoidance patterns are learnt from early childhood. We consciously steer clear of difficult situations by avoiding them. When we sense something difficult coming our way, we get on guard.

For example, some people cannot take criticism, so if they sense that something of that nature may be going on, they change the subject. This is often encountered in helping and may be one of the elements that needs to be challenged. More generally in life, if two people tend to disagree with each other about a certain issue, they ultimately learn not to talk about it. In this way each avoids an uncomfortable situation. Why make life complicated when it can be simple by avoiding certain people or problems?

Egan (1994, p. 313) talks about 'entropy', or inertia, as 'the human tendency to put off problem-managing action'. Laziness would probably mean that clients never actually get to be clients; they are too lazy to bother at all. Entropy prevents clients from grappling with a problem once they have recognized it. Clients resist being challenged; they suddenly declare that they feel tired; they tell you that they should not really have bothered you – or use some such tactic. Entropy is easily spotted but less easily acknowledged.

All blockages to growth are difficult to deal with. The most helpful way may be to treat them positively and work with them, rather than against them. They are in themselves negative and often destructive and it is easy to get hooked into them. The danger is that inexperienced helpers concentrate on the problem and so facilitate such blockages to thrive. The classic example is when a helper tries to find more and more possible ways of coping and each time the client replies, 'Yes, but...'. The skill is to concentrate on the person, not the problem.

Challenging

The whole of the helping process is a challenge. If clients were not stuck they would not seek help. But because they are stuck, they need help in getting out of that situation. This is possible only when they acknowledge that an attitude or behaviour has to be challenged. Because they cannot do this themselves, they need the challenge to come from outside. They are challenged by the process of helping, and they are challenging themselves to change.

To challenge another person well is a skill. But it is not just one specific skill. It is a composite of many helping skills and tactics in such a way that clients are gently pushed, pulled or prodded. Any challenge is *for* the client, and only with the client's goal in mind. Challenge should be positive; it is never meant for punishing.

But challenge does have something negative about it, therefore it should first of all reinforce. The person's strengths rather than weaknesses should be challenged. Such strengths, resources and assets need to be pointed out and addressed as they may not otherwise be fully recognized. They are, however, absolutely essential if the client's self-responsibility and self-helping skills are to be effective. Clients are challenged and helped to challenge themselves.

Any challenge should be concrete and specific. Simply to say 'You need to become more assertive' is not enough.

The manner in which a challenge is offered is very important. A challenge has to be based on some fact that the helper has observed. This can be an observation of body language or something that was said:

You say you are feeling fine but you look as though you are worried. I noticed that you said three times that you are not angry with him and I wonder whether this is really true because there seems to be a lot of anger between you which might not be expressed.
From what you say it seems that you have not looked at this aspect very carefully. Perhaps it isn't easy, but should you give it some thought now?

Challenge should be appropriate to the person concerned. Giving a challenge too hesitantly means that it may not be taken seriously enough. But giving it brutally may destroy a relationship and may also destroy a client who might be at a crucial moment of insight.

On the other hand it is also true, but perhaps sometimes not taken seriously enough by counsellors, that people are robust and can take a challenge. They often ask for it; they need it, but always with the aim of moving forward to self-help and self-challenge.

When there is a reason to challenge, your professional integrity demands that you do it. If you do not do it, clients may not be able to develop and may remain in the morass and perhaps even sink further into it.

One way of using challenging as a skill is with the 'sandwich technique': first you give praise or reinforcement – one slice

of bread. Then you give the challenge: the important filling.
Then you give more reinforcement or praise: the other slice
of bread.

Patient: Sally is home this week and we got on really well for the first
three days. But yesterday I lost my temper again. I just don't
seem to be able to get it right.

Nurse: You managed so well for three days, congratulations! Tell me
what you think made you lose your temper.

Patient: (describes in detail)

Nurse: You had three good days and that is more than you ever had
so far. You have also been together longer now than you had
managed before. I think your goal was realistic, but you have
gone back to that 'poor me' attitude which we talked about
before. Perhaps we need to consider it again. But start by giving yourself a pat on the back for having succeeded for
three days.

One reason for having a supervisor for your counselling and
helping is so that all aspects of your work can be discussed
and scrutinized. Helpers are as human as their clients, and so
also have blind spots, outmoded attitudes and self-defeating
behaviours. The question 'What is happening?' applies equally
to you as to your clients when work gets tough or when you
are dealing with particularly difficult patients and clients. It
would be paradoxical to challenge others unless you also challenge yourself in the way you live and work. When clients see
that their helpers are challengeable they may accept challenge
from them more easily.

Confronting with reality

When some blind spot is challenged the person can see the
reality of the world as it really is at that point, whereas before
it was distorted by behaviours and rules that had become the
inner driving force.

Confronting clients with reality in a helping relationship is
part of the skill of challenging. It is one aspect of helping them
to challenge themselves and develop new perspectives. Helpers who have a good understanding of the context of the client's world will clearly be more perceptive and able to help.
Those who help bereaved people need to have some understanding of bereavement; those who help children need to
have a good 'feel' for the world of children. Nurses are therefore in a very good position to help patients because both parties are in the environment that shapes them. This does not
yet mean that nurses can necessarily empathize with patients'

pain, fear or experience of loss. If nurses can learn from their patients and clients what it is like in their world, they are more likely to help them perceptively and accurately.

A very simple and perhaps even obvious example of the discrepancies exhibited by patients is shown in this extract from a conversation. The patient was brought into the present reality by the nurse confronting her in a reflective and empathic way:

Patient: No really, I'm fine.
Nurse: You are fine as far as your health is concerned, but you are sitting so tightly in the corner of your chair. You look as if you have a lot of pain inside yourself.
Patient: (loosening herself and after a long moment) I do have pain. . . It's the anniversary of my mother's death, and she had cancer too.

The following is from a personal journal of a nurse:

At first he talked and talked, and I listened, and in fact I would not have been able to get a word in edgeways. I was aware that I was listening without being reflective, and so, little by little, I started to reflect some of the things back to him in a digested way. I felt I had to feed him a bit of the reality of what is happening to other patients with his sort of condition. I said that when he was admitted his behaviour was very much that of letting us know that here comes A. He had to prove to us that he was still himself, that he was normal, and that he was going to kick against anything that was in any way abnormal. I felt that having said that, this was like a reassurance to him that he is in fact normal, that he has progressed since then, that we had accepted him as he was then, and as he is now, and also that we care about him. I felt that by giving him little bits of himself at a time, and by reflecting back what he had just given me in the way of information, I was able to confront him with the reality appropriate to him.

The question 'What is happening?' may be particularly useful at such moments as it may help to reveal the reality relevant to this moment in a person's life, and so help to acknowledge and adopt it for a more satisfying life-style.

The other skills mentioned in this chapter are all skills of challenging. They challenge clients to challenge themselves. This means that the skills that clients need to bring to a helping relationship are basically a willingness to collaborate in developing the 'handles' needed to change the current problems and emotional states.

Expressing feelings   When blocks exist that hinder growth and change, one way into or through the block is not to concentrate on the problem, but on the person. The way to reach the person is mainly by addressing the feelings present. But clients are often unsure of what their feelings are and need to be helped to express them realistically. In Chapter 8 the heading was 'Experiencing feelings' and the next chapter will consider 'Managing feelings'. Experiencing, expressing and managing feelings is all part of the same process, but this is divided here in order to facilitate the discussion.

Many people have difficulty in expressing their feelings. They may either not know how to do it well, or, if they do not feel safe, they dare not. Clients are vulnerable people if they are sick or well, and each aspect poses its own difficulties. Since feelings are the gateway to helping, it is important that they can be expressed and that clients do not feel judged, but supported and surrounded by empathy, warmth and genuineness from their helpers.

Nelson-Jones (1993, p. 320) suggests that, in order to express feelings, clients should be helped to focus both on thinking skills and action skills. Among the thinking skills he details the need to help clients know that they have a *choice* in expressing feelings; that they can *coach* themselves in statements like 'stay calm... speak firmly...' etc; that *realistic rules* concerning relationships should be chosen ('children should be seen and not heard' is an unrealistic rule); that more accurate *perceptions* of feelings should be developed; that clients should learn to *predict* more accurately other people's feelings concerning themselves. This last point is particularly pertinent as many people work on a basis of 'I have to get this right or she will be cross with me', meaning 'I have to conform to her needs in order to have a quiet life'. Such projections are very common and often false as clients twist themselves emotionally to the whims of others, when these whims may not even exist. It may take quite a while, though, for clients to see that this is their behaviour, take responsibility for it, and be able to change it.

The action skills that Nelson-Jones (1993, p. 322) mentions should concentrate on verbal, voice and body messages: what is said, how it is said and how it comes across.

A part-time care assistant was fond of a person she went to bath regularly in a sheltered flat. This person was partly paralysed and had a speech difficulty. The care assistant challenged her client one day by saying that she was never sure whether she was really welcome because the client's greeting was rather lukewarm. The client was surprised at this and together they considered what had led to the perceptions of each. The client had never given any thought to welcoming her friends, but the care assistant felt taken for granted. She suggested that the client put some enthusiasm into her voice when greeting her. They practised a couple of times to see what each of them understood this to mean. After a few weeks several of the client's friends commented on the change. The care assistant found herself taken aback once or twice by the change and the delightful difference it made. She told her client more than once how nice it was to be greeted in this warm way.

With the bad press that feelings often have it is not surprising that people find them difficult to deal with. But feelings are not some entity apart from us: they *are* us. As the helping relationship is usually concerned mainly with feelings, learning to experience and express them is often part of the work done in the relationship. Where better to learn about experiencing and expressing feelings than in a safe environment and with a supportive helper? The skill of immediacy is therefore the most obvious one to use in taking this aspect further.

Expressing feelings is not just an aspect of long-term counselling: in very short interactions some helping can often be done which highlights this aspect of caring. Indeed, many patients may be able to cope only with short interactions at more frequent intervals. The skill is therefore needed at every level of competence.

Immediacy

Most difficulties in most people's lives are those caused by interpersonal relationships. It is therefore quite likely that the difficulties that clients present are those that are to do with their relationships. Not surprisingly, this may be mirrored in the relationship with you as helper. Using the skill of immediacy may be a very powerful way of introducing this particular reality.

The skill of immediacy, or direct, mutual talk, or even 'you–me talk' (Egan, 1977) is particularly useful when there is some obvious – to you – mirroring taking place.

The mother of three teenage boys was in hospital having badly broken a leg falling off a chair while cleaning the windows of her house. The 15-year-old son had visited the night before but they had quarrelled.

Patient: This is all we do at home. We say little to each other and every conversation ends in one of us saying something wrong and then we fall into silence.

Nurse: Well, I have noticed that the talks between you and I seem to be 'on and off': sometimes we get on well and then we talk a bit and there is more silence than talk. We don't seem to know what to say to each other. I wonder if this is a bit like the conversations with your son?

Patient: You are right, you know. I seem to get stuck very easily with other people.

Nurse: Perhaps there is something in this which might shed some light on what is going on between you and those close to you.

This type of challenge, involving the helper in a more personal aspect, can be used to make comparisons of behaviour and perhaps point out to clients certain aspects of behaviour that might otherwise go unobserved or be difficult to challenge.

The following conversation took place between a patient and the breast-care nurse after the patient had had a mastectomy. The nurse was an experienced counsellor and this interaction shows not only immediacy, but particularly empathy, reflecting and clarifying, and general skills of communicating:

Patient: We've never had a marvellous sex life, but just now when I most need to feel I am still a woman he (her husband) is now totally impotent.

Nurse: You mentioned having to feel like a woman before; what does this actually mean to you?

Patient: I think you are not taking me seriously. I am asking you to help me with his impotence.

Nurse: Can I stop here for a moment and actually look at what is going on between us two?

Patient: Well, go on then.

Nurse: As I just said, you mentioned several times having to feel like a woman, and each time I asked you to think about it you switched the conversation away from you. I feel that you are asking for something but then refuse it when it is offered. I am actually feeling impotent to help you – or perhaps more strongly, I feel made impotent.

Patient: Are you saying that I am making my husband impotent?

Nurse: Not exactly. What I am saying is that our relationship here may very well mirror something that is going on at home.

Patient: I don't quite follow you.

Nurse: I feel that your relationship with your husband may have some element in it which is similar to your relationship with me. You may be asking something of him but, when he tries to give it to you, you don't accept it.

Patient: But you are not my husband.

Nurse: No, but I am picking up a similar way of behaving.
Patient: What am I asking from him then?
Nurse: You are asking from him how you can be a woman.
Patient: And he doesn't help me by being impotent.
Nurse: You are asking me, too, how can you be a woman?
Patient: Yes?
Nurse: How can you be a woman?
Patient: Well, how?
Nurse: Stay with that question for a while.
Patient: I don't know whether I can cope with this now.
Nurse: I expect that for you 'being a woman' is something far more important than the words might convey. I am pushing you now to look at that side of it, and perhaps your husband is pushing you in the same way to look at yourself, because you actually ask for it. What do you feel when I push you in this way?
Patient: Go away! It's rather hot!
Nurse: How does that tie in with your husband's 'going away'?

The relationship between helper and client becomes a model, and a place for trying out new behaviours. In what way is the relationship between helper and client different from the problematic one? What does this one have that the other does not? What is better here than there?

Egan (1994, p. 108) writes about empathy from different aspects and mentions in particular the communication skills aspect of it. He sees communication to have three dimensions:

Perceptiveness
Know-how
Assertiveness.

In the example above these are evident in the fact that the helper was perceptive in that she related her own feeling of impotence to that of her client: she felt unable to function adequately. Her know-how was shown in that she knew when to intervene and in a way that the client could understand. The client showed a great deal of resistance to understanding, but that is the nature of blind spots and blockages. The assertiveness of the helper was then shown in the way in which she stuck with her intervention and did not retaliate or answer in an aggressive way.

This client asked the counsellor basically to sort out her husband's problem. Sometimes clients think that if you can tell them what a third person should do, or say, the situation will improve. You cannot 'counsel' a third person, or effect a change in that person. You cannot even change the client. You can *help* clients to change themselves, and clients can then influence the relationship with that third person in the way that is most appropriate.

Self-sharing

Self-sharing is described here as one of the skills of challenging. It involves sharing something with the client in order to reassure, or to stimulate.

Many people feel very isolated with their feelings and think that they alone in the whole wide world suffer the particular problem and that nobody can understand them. It is possible gently to undo these assumptions by telling the client something about yourself and bringing a better reality into the situation.

Yes, I was once in a similar situation to you, and I can remember feeling almost the same as you are saying now: a feeling of loneliness and of being abandoned. It is difficult to feel like that and I can appreciate it, but this is not all there is to you. This is only one aspect and you have reason to believe that tomorrow it will be different.

One difficulty with self-sharing is that it can become 'I know exactly how you feel'. With the best empathy in the world you will never know *exactly* how someone else feels. A mother of a stillborn baby or a bereaved person might be particularly hurt by such a statement.

Self-sharing can also be done at a deeper level:

Nurse: As you are saying this I have a sense of being gripped by the throat. I would have found it difficult to be in that situation myself and I value what you told me here. Was it difficult for you to tell me?

Patient: I needed to tell it and get it out. I felt my throat being gripped when I thought about telling you. I am glad I did.

The experience of really being heard as a person is something that is often alien to clients. It can therefore be very important in expressing the value of being human for both people when such sharing can take place.

Self-sharing is often useful as a skill to challenge clients to look more clearly at either a feeling or an attitude. Such self-sharing is done with empathy:

Patient: I always say the wrong thing at the wrong time.

Nurse: I have so often felt like that too! I always feel such a fool then, and I guess that is how you are feeling too.

Clients can see helpers, including nurses, as experts and

thus 'above' them. Self-sharing is then tremendously liberating for both people. Suddenly you feel equals, two human beings with each other. But the aim of self-sharing is not that *you* feel better, but that your client can move forward. Self-sharing is a skill like the others because it has to be used with care: too much and you are in danger of loading your own burdens on to your client; too little and you may appear distant. As always, the skill is using it at the right time and in the right quantity, with the right kind of empathy.

Intuition

One form of self-sharing is the use of intuition. This can apply to all areas of helping: the client, the relationship, yourself, or to subconscious material that can be reached only by this 'sixth sense'.

As helper, you are deeply involved with your clients. But whereas clients are stuck, you are not. You see possibilities for moving forward. You make connections where clients have not done so. You see patterns that clients are blind to. These can help clients to see a wider picture. The skill lies in the way you present these pictures from your view so that they broaden the view that clients already have, rather than blot it out.

A hunch, an insight, an intuition is 'an involuntary event, which depends upon different external or internal circumstances, instead of an act of judgement'. (Jung, 1964, p. 49)

Ferrucci (1982, p. 222) puts this in a practical way:

Intuition perceives wholes, *while our everyday analytical mind is used to dealing with* parts *and therefore finds the synthesizing grasp of the intuition unfamiliar. But after an intuition does appear, it may even seem to us to have revealed something obvious; we ask, 'why haven't I seen this before?'*

When you use your intuition for helping it becomes a challenge. The client is jolted out of a narrow view of the self and the surrounding world into a wider view and into this 'whole' that has become available. Bridges may suddenly appear where there were none before and this may enable the person also to cross them.

Intuition is not only a helper skill; clients use it too. Helping goes on beyond the time spent with a person. When each has been opened to awareness, all sorts of places, words, pictures and dreams may give insights, and intuitively reveal the self to the self.

As a helper you may or may not be at ease with intuition. It is impossible to describe a 'technique' for using intuition. The only way to learn it is to listen. Ferrucci (1982, p. 224) goes on to say:

We can increase our intuitive capacity if we will acknowledge the possibility of our receiving intuitions, recognize their value, cherish them when they come, and finally, learn to trust them.

Helpers who use intuition 'naturally' cannot analyse too much what it is that they use, or why. When they recognize an insight or a hunch, they simply use it as part of their way of working. But those to whom it does not come naturally should not contrive it.

Intuitions or hunches can summarize a particular situation, throw new light on a problem, or enable fresh material to come to the surface. The use of intuition is a skill at one level, and at another level it is something subjective that 'happens'. Both aspects are valid when they are used for helping clients.

Sensation *(i.e. sense perception) tells you that something exists;* thinking *tells you what it is;* feeling *tells you whether it is agreeable or not;* and intuition *tells you whence it comes and where it is going.* (Jung, 1964, p. 49)

This means therefore that intuition can be helpful at all stages of helping but particularly when goals are being shaped.

Empowering

Empowering has become a politically correct word and has therefore lost some of its possible impact. What all helping is intending to do, however, is to empower the clients. This means that, at the end of a helping relationship, clients are able to function more satisfyingly and resourcefully than before. This could also be described as positive living or creative living (Dowrick, 1993).

Some of the blockages to change described above are strategies to remain powerless. It can be so easy to blame parents, the government, fate, God – anything and anyone – for a particular state of affairs. Those who do not use such tactics tend to think that a person is just plain lazy, and they may be right. Those who are achievers might point to discipline as a means to getting somewhere. Others might point to a belief in the self as the answer. They may all be right. But as helpers we do not have a mandate to tell our clients what they must do or think or how they must behave. We can only help clients to find the goals to which they themselves aspire and to find the means to achieving them which lie within themselves. The empowering needs to happen so that goals can be sought, but more importantly the clients must be keen to put them into action by wanting to change.

In the process of change there are three important steps:

Awareness
Acknowledgement
Change.

Clients become clients because they are aware that something is not as it should be, but they are usually not able to say what this 'something' is. Through the help given in assessing the situation and the problem, they come to the point of being able to name the problem. This means usually working *with* blockages and blind spots rather than against them or through them. Through exploring and challenging, clients come to the insights that lead to understanding and meaning and acknowledgement. Only when this has happened – and it need not be a dramatic experience – can the change take place. We cannot change if we do not know what to change.

Like all processes, helping goes through a phase of introspection, which often means admitting some form of powerlessness. It seems as if we need to reach a nadir so as to see the zenith.

Challenging is part of this process. Because the emphasis should be on challenging strengths rather than weaknesses, this is legitimate. Challenging the strengths is empowering.

Clients will often say, 'Why had I not seen this before?' My answer to this is usually that they had not been ready for it before. The help given them by talking with a person who does not judge and who has only their good in mind will gradually have brought to the surface material that had been subconscious and even unconscious. But first of all the material had to come to the awareness. Then it had to be acknowledged. Only then could it be changed.

The whole of the helping process is a challenge. But it is so because the clients are willing to be challenged and to challenge themselves. They are helped in this by counselling skills. The aim of counselling is that clients are able to help themselves; if clients become dependent on counsellors there is a potential difficulty and clearly there is no empowering.

When the helping process has been successful, clients are ready to move forward and outward. The most empowering thing that helpers may then be able to say to them is: 'Go on then, do it'. This is more than simply a permission, as the permission to talk was given at the beginning of the process. It is now rather a confirmation that the process has been successful and the helper trusts the client implicitly to do what needs to be done. This trust was there from the beginning, but at the end it is perhaps the greatest gift that helpers can give to their clients. It is that which enables and empowers them to trust in themselves in a way that is liberating.

CHAPTER 10

Client skills: goal setting

Client skills

The process of counselling and helping is for the clients. The skilled helper can do so much, but clients need to do the rest.

As so often in describing skills and helping relationships, it is difficult to describe only one facet and not the many others that are also present. But such is the limitation of the printed page... This chapter describes some of the skills that clients should be able to acquire during a helping relationship. The helper's skills described in the two preceding chapters should have enabled this to happen.

This does not mean teaching clients new tricks, though some of the ways of coping may be new to clients. It is a question of helping clients to weigh up strengths and weaknesses and to build on their strengths in order to compensate for and overcome the weaknesses. The basic skill for both clients and helpers is a collaboration which will have been demonstrated by helpers as active listening, reflecting, immediacy and self-sharing, and challenging.

New perspectives

To find the direction or goal in which to move, clients need to have various possibilities. To be effective as human beings, they have to make choices, and these are possible only when there are alternatives. The process of goal setting is thus a process of choosing from alternatives, or seeing the best way forward from among a variety.

In the story of the person in the ditch (see Chapter 6), the empathic helper has one foot in the ditch where the client is and keeps one foot on the firm ground. This conveys the image of a certain distance which may be needed at this stage. As helper you can step in closer to the client and step out to let the client help himself or herself as necessary. But you do not, in the image of this analogy, pull the client up by yourself. At best you can provide a ladder, or help the client to walk along the ditch to find the best way out by some steps that may be there, or a path, or some other way. By your support you help and guide the client to the way out which is meant for that particular person. You may give the client hints on how to look for these paths to better living; indeed, these hints may be the new perspectives that may come to light as you talk. Some of these hints use the subconscious and 'sixth sense', or perhaps latent psychic powers of both client and helper. With the helper skills described in preceding chapters and with empathy you may have noticed the strengths that clients have, and these can be used to good effect now.

Any analogy is useful when it helps to make a specific point but beyond that it shows its shortcomings: it is only an analogy and not the real thing. What matters is that clients are helped and can get to grips with their situation and change what needs to be changed. For new perspectives to be brought on to the scene now they have to draw on every resource. This can range widely. The danger is that helpers who are mostly thinking-oriented may neglect the feelings aspects of a situation, or those who are more in touch with feelings may neglect the thinking aspects. When you are aware of these pitfalls, you can be more open to what might present itself.

As helping involves the whole person, so the new perspectives should be as whole and holistic as possible. This means mind and body, spirit and matter, inner and outer, thinking and feeling, old and new, right and left brain, light and shadow – not in a dualistic fashion, but seeing opposites in order to integrate them. When helpers are able to do this, then clients are enabled to function more holistically as well. Helpers and clients can let their imagination roam as widely as possible.

Imagination

The helping skills outlined so far have concentrated on what is happening now and on what has gone before to bring a person to the present state. Essentially, helping is for the future: what life might be like from now on. That has to do with imagination. We cannot *know* the future; we can only imagine it. In the process of goal setting, this is the client's best tool for getting out of the ditch or rut and moving towards a better and more comfortable future. One of the first skills that clients can be helped to develop is therefore the imagination.

Many people feel that imagination is kids' stuff and that to be adult is to be rational. Rogers (1978, p. 99) quotes research on senior level managers which showed that the most effective and productive managers of enterprises were able to 'engage in personal fantasy, daydreams, fictional speculations . . . think and associate to ideas in unusual ways, have unconventional thought processes . . . (are) skilled in social techniques of imaginative play, pretending, and humour'.

Clients are stuck, or in a morass, precisely because they cannot imagine how to get out of it. If they did, they would not need help.

This may be the moment when an insight had been reached and the question 'What is the meaning of it?' had been answered. Inevitably, the next question is, 'Where do I go from here?' Sometimes there is a clear answer to this, but, when there is not, the imagination may come in useful.

Mary was the mother of 24-year-old Christopher with Down's syndrome. She had looked after him single-handedly since the death of her husband two years earlier. Christopher had another attack of bronchitis and Mary was afraid this would turn into pneumonia. The GP had visited and had also alerted the community nurse, who now called in without an appointment.

Mary: It's at times like this that I get down. I am totally tied up with him, and then I realize that I have no life of my own.

Nurse: You sound rather resentful.

Mary: You could say that.

Nurse: It's difficult never to do your own thing.

Mary: I've turned all the possibilities over and over in my mind and there is no solution that I would be happy with other than caring for him myself.

Nurse: There may not be a solution, but there may be some other things that could make your life easier.

Mary: What sort of things?

Nurse: What would your life be if it were just a little better? Not perfect, just a little better?

Mary: I would see more of my friends, get that degree . . .

This question asked Mary to use her imagination. Mary had always rejected sending Christopher to a home because she and her husband had always maintained that they should care for him. Since her husband's death in a car crash she felt her obligation even more strongly. She had one of those internal rules which maintained that she *must* care for him whatever happens. When the nurse asked her to imagine her world being better, this brought in some lateral thinking.

Notice also how the nurse addressed Mary and her life, not

the 'problem'. That opened the possibility to be imaginative rather than seeking a solution.

Imagination asks clients to think without constraint for a moment and to roam freely with their thoughts. The imagination can do wonders for clients who may see themselves on top of mountains, taking off on flying carpets or being as rich as Croesus. Many such images will never come true, but the fact that people stuck in a morass *can* let such images happen means that they have broken through some mindset that kept them hemmed in.

In the example above the nurse asked Mary to imagine what life might be like if it were 'a little' better. Between the sublime and the ridiculous there is often a middle way which may be found if the imagination can be tapped. Just daring to imagine that life can be different is often a first step. One patient, after having a colostomy raised, imagined she was a famous soprano. This was a very positive step for her on the road to recovery. She now sings in a local choir as a soprano. In her own eyes she is 'famous'; and indeed she is.

Imagination can be fostered in a great variety of situations.

Helper:	What would you have liked to have said to him?
Client:	I am not your servant.
Helper:	What could you change that you haven't changed so far?
Client:	I could go to work there on Tuesdays rather than Wednesdays.
Helper:	What decisions could you take now rather than wait?
Client:	I could make contact with her now, then I would know where I stand in relation to her to begin with.

The aim of helping is for clients to manage their life more resourcefully and satisfyingly. For this to happen, there needs to be some exploration and clarification. When clients can begin to use their imagination they are already able to see further than they had done before. There may have been little self-analysis until now. Once a person can imagine a direction, then self-analysis will happen 'by the way'. Imagination can be not only vital for this, but also refreshingly new, and fun.

Visualization

A close partner to imagination is visualization. This is a practical skill that is often associated with meditation. It has been widely used by Simonton et al. (1978) with patients who have cancer. Gawain (1978, p. 16) has made visualization much more widely applicable. She calls the basic steps in creative visualization:

1. Setting your goal.

2.   Creating a clear idea or picture.
3.   Focusing on it often.
4.   Giving it positive energy.

These steps are remarkably similar to the processes of helping and deciding. The principles are easily learned and applied. Gawain thinks that visualizing better relationships could change lives dramatically. Clients who have particular difficulties with a relationship can be encouraged to use visualization as a possibility in the search for a way forward.

When it has emerged what the particular problem is with a relationship, clients can be encouraged to use visualization.

Client: I just cannot get through to her.
Nurse: 'Getting through to her' is your goal here?
Client: At least as a start.
Nurse: If you hold her in your mind's eye now, try to see her just as the person she is. Try now to see a clear channel of light between her and you, with both of you communicating, and with you getting through to her. Keep this picture in mind and repeat it as often as you can in the day. Once the picture becomes 'alive' you can give it positive energy by thinking in terms of you loving her and she loving you, and both of you feeling close to each other. It takes some time for this to happen, but by repeating it you can change the energy field between you.

The helper may know of the technique and how it is applied, but the client has to carry out the visualization and be willing to do it and permit the results to cause change.

Although this technique works particularly well with relationships, it is useful for many situations where a change of attitude is desired, such as in wanting to let go of inner rules and outdated values. The technique is there to see oneself in the positive light without that rule or that heavy baggage, for as long as is needed.

Managing feelings

Since much emphasis is placed on feelings in helping, one outcome of helping must be that clients can manage their feelings better than before. Feelings are not some entity but are part of ourselves. This means in essence that managing feelings is managing ourselves. What often happens is that clients will ask for help with one particular feeling and other feelings, perhaps more strongly felt ones, come to the fore. But when one feeling is managed better, then it is also possible that the others can be. The goal may therefore be to concentrate on one feeling, or one aspect of a feeling, to begin with.

Nelson-Jones (1993, p. 323) advocates that the management of feelings is best done by concentrating on thinking skills and action skills. He describes three main types of feelings: anger, depression and anxiety. Each of these feelings has different thinking skills, though the thinking skill that remains the same for all three is 'possessing realistic personal rules'. The other thinking skills consist of owning responsibility for anger and perceiving self and others accurately in anxious situations. Self-instruction and visualization are also considered thinking skills. The action skills for anger concentrate mainly on assertion, such as expressing anger, requesting behavioural changes and handling aggressive criticism. The action skills for anxiety need to be considered differently for each specific situation.

The other thinking skills for depression mentioned by Nelson-Jones (1993, p. 324) are 'perceiving others and self accurately', 'attributing (the) cause accurately' and 'predicting realistically'. The action skills here are also concerned with assertion, but also with relationship skills and pleasant activities. Barker (1993) has not divided the skills into such clear categories, but in his *A Self-Help Guide to Managing Depression* he outlines very similar tactics.

Since the skills for goal setting are essentially the client's own skills, perhaps helped into existence by a counsellor or helper, it is useful to consider tactics which may be simple but effective.

One of the best starting points for managing any feelings is to consider the personal rules that clients have. So often these rules are unrealistic and so deeply embedded that it is difficult to recognize them. The age-old question that many patients ask themselves and their nurses is, 'Why me?' They cannot believe that bad things should happen to them when they have been trying so hard all their lives to be 'good', perhaps not smoking, not eating meat, and so on. We have all seen such situations; the following one simply sums them up:

We were on holiday and I suddenly had this flutter in my chest and I could not feel a real pulse. They soon put it right in hospital, but I simply cannot understand why this should have happened when I have been alright for five years now after the operation. It has left me so weak, and of course we had to abandon the holiday.

This patient could not take in that his holiday should be disrupted by arrhythmia when he had booked the holiday specially to go walking and thus keep fit. It was inconceivable that his plans were disrupted. How dare this happen to him! Such rules help us to get through life, but when they become too inflexible or unrealistic, they cause trouble. Although this patient never mentioned anger, this was the underlying feeling and he was helped to experience this, and express it. When he learnt how to think about this personal rule, he discovered a whole host of other such rules. By concentrating on this one first, he managed to get the others into some perspective which eventually allowed him to live life in a more relaxed mode.

Managing resistance

Resistance is often a defence mechanism or a trade-off for negative feelings. If clients fear that they may be censured or judged, they will resist helpers. This can happen at any point in the helping process. If there is the slightest pressure by helpers to focus on anything specific, or to move towards a goal that will need some change, a resistance builds up. This may be part of a usual pattern and be the cause of the problem. It may also simply be a by-product of the process. It is clearly an important factor in relationships when a client has been sent to a counsellor, such as in schools, the probation service and in psychiatry. Helpers can cut through much of this with a non-judgemental attitude and by giving permission to talk and to acknowledge the resistance.

When clients have become aware of their resistance, they may want to find ways in which to help themselves deal with the problem. It is again Nelson-Jones (1993) who suggests that resistance can be managed with the two-fold approach of thinking skills and action skills.

The first skill mentioned by Nelson-Jones (1993, p. 142) is that of owning responsibility for choosing. Clients who have come to an understanding about meaning earlier in the process will see more easily how this skill applies to them. The need for 'personalising the experience' (Carkhuff) exists in order to own feelings in the first instance. In the same way, 'I statements' help to get in touch with what is really happening. Throughout the helping process there is thus an emphasis on owning responsibility. This does not mean that clients shoulder the burden of everything around them. On the contrary, by learning to own responsibility for themselves, they are likely to learn also what and who else also has responsibility, and to leave that responsibility to them. Realistic personal rules are therefore also important. This is another of the thinking skills advocated here.

The action skills demand a fair degree of commitment from clients. Those who have been working towards goals are already clearly well on the way. For others it may be more difficult. The helper's constant support and challenge where necessary complement the process.

Action skills really mean action here: doing something which shows that resistance can be overcome. This may mean taking a first, and perhaps small, step in the right direction, just so that it is clear that resistance can be overcome and be an incentive to be more daring and more assertive. For many people this is not some great plan, but perhaps making a telephone call, or writing a letter that had been put off. For patients and clients it may also mean asking a dreaded question; negotiating for time to think further about a treatment option before deciding; or deciding to make a complaint rather than go on suffering.

I used to give my friends the impression that I was very self-sufficient, I think. Until I got ill. Then they told me that I must do this, go to that doctor, not be so stubborn. For a while I enjoyed this care and began to feel very fragile. When all the tests turned out to be negative I realized with one great leap that I have to trust my intuition. I knew what was the matter with me, but a doctor would not be able to help me with this. My pain was emotional pain. What a laborious way to learn it. I could not show my feelings, but being taken over and really manipulated by my friends brought out my feelings alright! The question was then how not to blame them. I think I have managed to do this reasonably well.

The way in which resistance is managed depends on the kind of goals envisaged and set, and is part of the process of goal setting.

Goal setting

Having to think of and working towards formulating goals focuses the attention, mobilizes energy, increases persistence, and motivates clients to search for strategies (Egan, 1994, p. 221).

The question 'What is your goal?' is very specific and the answer to it should also be specific. The whole of helping should have led to such a position. While clients search for goals, helpers need to encourage them in goal-finding and goal-stating; hence the need for the helper skills of clarifying, focusing and shaping. A sense of direction and versatility in clients and helpers are the main aspects of goal setting.

The whole of the helping process has been geared towards a goal and therefore to change. That goal and that change need to be expressed now in terms that are specific and have a tangible outcome.

If the challenging has been done well by helpers, then clients will come to a goal. Helpers may therefore have needed to ask 'What is your goal?' many times and coached clients in self-help possibilities.

Egan (1994) emphasizes again and again that goals must have some results, that is, goals must be stated in terms of accomplishments rather than just programmes or activities. Clients should first of all believe that a goal is worthwhile, and then see it already as a reality. The principle of setting objectives for any task can be applied here. For example:

After reading this book nurses and helpers will use counselling skills effectively at work.
When I leave hospital I will have practised looking at my wound.
In a year's time from now I will have written the first essay in my degree course. (See above, the mother of Christopher.)

A goal need not be just one particular thing. A goal can be one main aim with different means of achieving it. It can be a main goal with several smaller goals set before it. It can be two or three goals, each depending on the other. There are many ways of thinking of goals and of taking action to reach them. What matters is that they are clearly stated and make sense to clients.

It may be that a client has as an overall goal a statement like, 'I want to become a more assertive person'. But this has to be stated in practical terms. This may be something like, 'In two weeks (give the date) I want to have contacted my brother about that missing file; if he does not answer within three weeks I will write again. In a month I will have read that book about assertiveness. In three months I will have tried five exercises from the book'.

Goals need above all to be realistic. If too much is aimed for then the first attempt will bring disaster. If too little is aimed at then it may not even be worthwhile trying. What is realistic may need to be checked out with the helper because the reasons for seeking help in the first instance – the blind spots, inconsistencies and defence mechanisms – may show themselves again and still influence the thinking and acting at this stage.

You may need to help your clients to change an intention into a detailed and distinctive goal, 'I will spend two evenings a week with the children', rather than leaving it as, 'I must spend more time with the children'.

When a goal is clear and specific in this way it can be measured or evaluated. At the end of the week the client can look back and see whether two evenings were indeed spent with the children. If it was not possible, the reason can be established. Was it due to outside influences beyond control, or was it again work (the problem) which got in the way? If it was, was the goal realistic?

Client: I want to be with my children but I also love my work.
Helper: Which do you really love more?
Client: Work fulfils me in a way that home doesn't.
Helper: So you stay on at work and don't get home when they expect you.
Client: Work never finishes in a hospital, you know that too, and I feel needed there . . .
Helper: How realistic then is it for you to have two evenings at home?
Client: I should be able to fit it in.
Helper: You *should*
Client: I also *want* to.
Helper: And *can* you?
Client: I could if I tried. I'll give it another go. No, wait a minute: two evenings one week, one evening the next. That will give me a bit more leeway and will allow me to try it out more.

Revising a goal is not necessarily a step backwards. It may be a more realistic step forward. In this case the client had the idea of a 'compromise' with himself. This shows both thinking and action skills based on realistic personal rules. Such self-responsibility leads to a sense of direction and versatility which may ultimately be more important than keeping to a predetermined plan. It also shows that this client was well on the way to using self-help skills and therefore felt himself to be more in control of his life and attitudes.

Some people learn only by their mistakes, and to make mistakes can be important. It can also be very painful, particularly after having gone through a process or period of counselling. Having set realistic goals, it is also important to avoid as many pitfalls as possible by realistic planning.

Planning for change

There is no shortage of expressions to describe what is now the next step. Every model of helping and management has some way of describing the crucial step from a mental to a practical activity. Plans and strategies have to be 'translatable' from one sphere to another. This is again something that clients have to do themselves, but with the support of helpers.

The best support that helpers can give at this moment is stimulating the client's existing skills and knowledge. As a helper you are never a complete step ahead of the client, but you are nevertheless a little ahead in that you are not in the same position. Your own personal experience and that of other clients you have helped will give you the advantage of being able to suggest possible strategies. When these possibilities are presented to clients they are able to see which may fit or not fit and which may be 'do-able' or not. But most of all, they may also stimulate further and different possibilities that may so far have been hidden.

Just as values are chosen, prized and acted on (see Chapter 4), so the same has to happen with goals: once the goal has been chosen it has to be prized in the sense that it must be valued and considered carefully with a view to being put into action. If a goal is not valued enough, it cannot be put into action in a way that is valuable and adds value to the client's life.

The strategies that are developed have to do with coping and overcoming blocks and resistances. They have therefore to be kind but firm, challenging but exciting, difficult but also simple, different but also familiar. Trying to change the world overnight is not very helpful.

Some clients may know exactly what they want and need, and once stated, they go and make the necessary changes. Others may need a good deal of coaxing and stimulating before they can begin to state how they might put something into action. The question 'How are you going to do it?' may – like all the other questions – have to be asked several times before a realistic answer can be found and given.

The shy or unassertive patient who says, 'I have to speak to the consultant about it' may need to be asked, 'How might you ask him?' This question may help the client to formulate her own question in such a way that she will stick to it and not be flustered when the consultant turns up in a hurry.

'How are you going to do it?' is a question that addresses the client's own capacities for acting. It is not just a question that helpers ask their clients, but is above all the question that clients can ask themselves and need to answer for themselves.

Depending on the type of goal, there are plenty of practical means of 'seeing' the strategies:

Brainstorming.
Force-field analysis.
Making lists.
Looking for incentives and rewards.
Asking for specific advice from experts.

Strategies, or the means of achieving goals, can be as varied as the goals and, when clients have been helped to be more self-responsible, they may also be more imaginative and generate their own ideas for finding strategies. These may correspond to the client's personality type and therefore come easy, or they may also look to challenge such types. For instance, a 'thinking' person may deliberately want to look at strategies in the way a more 'feeling' person would do, so as to get to grips with such ways of acting.

This sounds rather 'heavy' and more concerned with long-term counselling. But the method is exactly the same for short and one-off situations. The concepts are then reduced and there is much less deliberation involved. Once the basic Four Questions have been asked and answered – though not necessarily as these particular questions – the process will have been gone through.

Egan (1994, p. 315) says that at this stage clients should have become effective tacticians. He defines *tactics* as 'the art of adapting a plan to the immediate situation'. This means a capacity to combine vision and praxis in such a way that the outcome is pleasing and useful. It may mean being flexible and open-minded, but also very determined. Helpers who have been effective will have done much to give their clients the necessary confidence to use their skills in these ways.

A moral contract

When a client and helper have worked together on a problem, it is not only helpful but necessary for them to finish this work in a way that enhances them both.

For a person to have admitted to a difficulty in front of another can sometimes be painful and is often significant. Something 'unmentionable' spelled out is a form of getting rid of it. Talking about it is cleansing. It is also a kind of commitment to carry out what has been talked about. The issue is now not any longer only in the mind of one person; it is shared. Two people are now involved. There is therefore a moral 'contract' as well as a practical one. This may sometimes have to be pointed out.

Having such a contract is more than the nuts and bolts of meeting. It is also more than simply being kind and telling the helper of the successes achieved, showing what a good client he or she was by doing what had been promised. It is an inner commitment to the self, the other and the relationship. Helping is about being and becoming more fully human, and the commitment is to human development as much as to the actual goal. Sometimes this may be spelled out, sometimes not. The quality of the relationship is often a good enough bond to keep to a unspoken contract.

The client skills described in this chapter are possible to realize only when the groundwork of helping and counselling has been done well. But the aim of such helping is for constructive change to take place. Only clients themselves can do the changing. They may not only want to change, but, at the end of a period of relating to someone who has their interests at heart, changing may also become a necessity which might not have been obvious before.

CHAPTER ELEVEN

Ending the relationship

....

Putting into action Once clients have reached the stage of applying their goals, they have reached a natural ending in the need for help. This should be acknowledged by both sides. If either helpers or clients are not ready to let go, there is a difficulty and this may have to be worked through.

There is something exciting about putting new plans into action. It opens horizons which may either not have been there, or which clients imagine might never have been for them. This may not be anything earth-shattering. Just the thought of approaching a problem from a different angle may be enough to change life for the better. Patients who might never have been aware of the psychological aspect of physical illness may feel much improved when a difficulty is either removed or reduced. The energy produced by the possibility of realistic change may alone be enough to make them better.

Some clients, on the other hand, consider change inevitable, to be endured rather than enjoyed. This may be particularly true for patients who have to come to terms with living with a disability or failing health, or indeed facing death. Accepting the inevitable may not be what they want most of all. But, they might argue, better to accept the inevitable because it cannot be changed. Trying to change their attitude and outlook may therefore be hard work.

While all of us helpers would prefer to see patients accepting the inevitable, this is far from usual. We cannot change others, and they may not want to be changed. Whatever we bring to a helping situation in the way of empathy and congruence can, by itself, bring about change, but we cannot rely on it. What we can rely on is the possibility that the unexpected may happen; that whatever does happen, happens at the right time and in the right way; and our own commitment to support clients whatever happens.

Setbacks

Even the best-laid plans will sometimes go wrong; even the most confident of persons has setbacks, which can be painful. When clients tell me that they had got on so well and then something happened that set them back, I often use the comparison with a waltz. The waltz has two steps forward and one step back, and both are necessary for the dance to go on. Setbacks can be seen like such a step backwards: they are necessary in order to go forward.

Setbacks can be very hurtful and bring clients back to points of pain which they thought they had put behind them.

Patient: I thought I had really forgiven my mother and we got on well for over a month. Then it was that remark from my daughter which opened up another can of worms and I seem to have fallen back even further. It was so humiliating.

The important thing here is to remember that this is not a setback of the 'snakes and ladders' type. It is not a game that is put right with a bit of luck. When clients have a sense of failure after a good run, they have moved forwards already. A setback is a new awareness. It is a new recognition of a situation which is now built on considerable experience since the last similar understanding. The image of a spiral can help: clients may find themselves on the same side of the spiral as before, but higher or lower on the depth-dimension. Thus the understanding of the present situation is now with more knowledge and insight, and certainly with more self-awareness.

When an old problem turns up again it is very likely that the patterns and blind spots, which had been at work before the helping intervention, are simply so deep that much more work needs to be done before they are no longer destructive. This needs long-term counselling from an experienced counsellor. There will always be patients and clients who have done a great deal of work on themselves with only minimal help, but when they need care or treatment from nurses they find that they need also counselling help to get them through a difficult time. This may then mean picking up the pieces at an advanced level of care: higher or lower in the spiral, depending on how one views the symbol. Such clients may be well aware of their problems but may also be looking for some quality help from nurses. For the clients the situation may present a setback; for nurses and helpers it may be a completely new problem.

If setbacks in the process of change are due to inattention, laziness or lack of discipline, this is more serious. It may then be that the goal was not serious enough or challenging enough, and this may mean going back over the process. Starting with the question 'What is happening?', it is possible for clients and helpers to review their work.

When setbacks are due to completely unexpected circumstances, it may mean that the earlier work may not have been done well. What is it about the present scenario that brought it to the surface? Was there something in the earlier work that had not been attended to? If so, new goals or perhaps new strategies might have to be considered and tried out.

Imagine that the client in the example in the last chapter, who wanted to ask the consultant some important question about herself but was very shy, found that she did not have the courage to do so at the time. This is clearly a setback and the strategy of rehearsing her line beforehand did not work. It may then be possible to consider new ways of helping the client to find the courage to ask her questions:

She may ask for the consultant to visit her specially and without his retinue so that she may feel less inhibited.
She may ask the nurse who had been helping her to be with her while she speaks to the consultant to give her moral support but not speaking for her.
She may ask to visit the consultant in a clinic.

These may not be first-line strategies but may be considered after a setback.

When setbacks happen it is very important that helpers support clients and do not punish. 'I told you so' is not helpful. Going back over the process and asking the Four Questions again is, however, constructive. The word 'setback' may not need to be used at all. Indeed, it may not be a failure on the part of the client, but more of a recognition and new awareness that all is not yet well and that more work might need to be done.

Self-monitoring

If clients are to put their goals into practice, then clearly they need to be able to monitor how this is working. The skill which they therefore need to acquire during a process of helping is to make sound judgements about themselves. Self-awareness and self-responsibility help towards the development of this skill, but most of us find it quite difficult to be objective about ourselves. We do not know whether we have done well or badly. Only from other people's reactions can we judge how we have done. When we become confident about something, we also become better judges about our skills.

Once the helping relationship is over, clients may still need ways and means of learning more. They now have to stand on their own and possibly without any support. They may ask you how to continue to learn on their own. The following strategies can be suggested to help them to monitor themselves. They can of course be used during a helping process as well as afterwards.

One of the difficulties that clients often display when judging themselves is that they tend to have different standards for themselves and for others. Many people judge themselves much more harshly than others. The 'realistic personal rules' show up as not being so realistic. They can forgive everyone else their faults but would never dream of forgiving themselves for theirs.

Self-monitoring is a skill that clients may need to learn in order to challenge their own unrealistic rules. Statements and slogans such as

Good enough is good enough.
I am responsible to, not for.
I have the same rights as everyone else.

may help in the learning of personal rules.

Many strategies for change may include checklists of goals achieved. This is a very visible way of self-monitoring. Much more difficult is knowing whether feelings were well experienced, expressed and managed. Among the self-help skills that clients may need to learn may first be the skill of monitoring themselves. Once this has been learnt, it is much easier to change other attitudes.

One popular way of self-monitoring is by keeping a journal or diary. This is not simply a log of the various activities of the day, but perhaps a diary of how feelings were experienced, how they were expressed and how they were managed. The beauty of diaries and journals is that they can be re-read and patterns can thus be detected. Nelson-Jones (1993, p. 285) describes two types of logs which correspond with his thinking and action skills model:

Stimulus, response and consequences logs:
Stimulus (what happened?)
Response (how I acted)
Consequences (what resulted?)
Situation, thoughts and consequences logs:
Situation (what happened and when?)
Thoughts (what I thought)
Consequences (how I felt and acted).

If a change has gone well, then it needs to be seen to have gone well and experienced as such. A goal exists, after all, to be achieved. Therefore it has to be measurable and achievable. At the other side of the goal, so to speak, it has to be experienced as having been worthwhile. When the goal has been well achieved, clients have to feel good about it. Helpers, too, may need to feel that their helping has been worthwhile. This is much more difficult to assess because contact with clients is often lost at the moment when a goal is transformed into action. Helpers, therefore, have also to have good self-monitoring skills.

Evaluation

Where at all possible, an evaluation of the helping process should take place. This may be a simple summary of what had been covered in a conversation, or it may be a complex review of a long-term relationship. If helping exists to enable clients to be in a better or more comfortable position than before, then this has to be acknowledged. Sometimes a simple question can help perform such an evaluation:

How do you feel now?
Where are you at now?
Where does this leave you now?

It can be useful for helpers to recapture the main points or difficulties covered and so show clients how much ground they have covered. This may be a way of reaffirming the work done and reaffirming the person. At the same time it is an encouragement to clients and may help to consolidate the path that they are now taking on their own.

For clients, an evaluation can be a time and occasion to show their self-help and self-monitoring skills. It may also be an opportunity for them to show their gratitude to helpers. Not that this is necessarily asked for, but clients may want and need to say 'thank you'. This is a need that has to be respected and can help to end the relationship in a really good way.

Ending the relationship

All of us know the situation where the most important thing in a conversation was said as the person was getting up from the chair or standing in the doorway. Ending a counselling session or process is as difficult and as important as beginning one.

Most of the counselling situations in nursing are short. Notable exceptions are those in mental health, the care of the elderly, and in community nursing. In these settings, where

relationships are long term, the ending may have to be prepared for and worked on. The severing of a long and perhaps
close personal tie may be like a death. For many patients this
may be repeating a process that they have already gone
through in relation to their own illness. If an important person
in their life now leaves as well, this may evoke the old pain.
Feelings of rejection by and hostility towards helpers may be
quite strong, and to some extent legitimate.

In more short-term situations there are other difficulties.
Patients and clients may on occasion feel ashamed that they
might have uncovered more about themselves than they were
initially prepared for. Or they may wonder why they 'burdened
that young girl' with their story in the first place. A simple
statement that it was you who encouraged them to do so may
be reassuring. It can also help to say to clients that you are
aware that this sort of talking may have made them uncomfortable. Confirmation that anything said between helpers and clients is confidential may also be helpful at the moment of ending.

People who say the most important thing when the time is
up have a reason for doing it in this way. They may not have
trusted themselves to talk about it before, or may have wanted
to test the helper out first to see whether she or he could be
trusted. It may be important at such a time to acknowledge
that you have heard the throw-away remark, but that the time
is now up. To indicate when you will be available again may
not only be polite, but may encourage a sense of security
and continuity.

It may sometimes be helpful in counselling to state shortly
before the end that there are only so many minutes left. This
can help clients to get their priorities in order at that moment.
Flexibility and firmness have to be combined in endings, as
do genuine care and challenge.

In the analogy of the victim in the ditch, both helper and
client are eventually on the road, on firm ground, needing to
go their separate ways. The purpose of helping is to let clients
find their own journey, and for them to be pleased to take it.

The person who teaches others to ride a bicycle, or to swim,
will sooner or later have to give them a push and then let go.
Perhaps the difference between sympathy and empathy is that
push. You say to the client, you *are* yourself, now *be* yourself.

One reason for supervision is that helpers sometimes have
blind spots about endings by denying how important people
are to them, and they to them. It may be as difficult for helpers
to let go as it is for clients. The awareness ('What is

happening?') and the point ('What is the meaning of it?') can lead to a redefinition ('What is my goal?') by being self-responsible and skilled ('What am I going to do about it?'). Clients and helpers have thus a responsibility to each other which may go further than meets the eye.

There may be many reasons for ending a helping relationship. Clearly, when a natural end has been reached there is no reason to continue in the role of helper and client. As the two people move through the process of helping, their relationship changes constantly. At the end it may not be a helper–client relationship so much as a partnership of equals negotiating space and needs. Both will have learned and changed; they will have needed each other, but they will also have given each other a new meaning in their lives. Helpers may forget their clients, but clients tend to remember their helpers.

CHAPTER TWELVE

Specific issues

··

This chapter considers a range of issues that have to be kept in mind by helpers. Some of them are more important for some people than for others. Depending on the setting and type of helping, some are present and some are not, or at least not strongly. They all concern the two people in the relationship but are mainly the domain of the helper.

Opportunities for using counselling skills

The daily life of a nurse is full of opportunities for helping in a counselling manner. What matters is the way in which you react to and deal with each opportunity.

Your role is first of all that of nurse, and you will probably be using counselling skills because you have realized that you are more effective in giving holistic care when you have that additional expertise. The distinction between counselling and using counselling skills (see Chapter 3) may sometimes be difficult and sometimes ideal. Only you will know which role you are more comfortable with.

When you are bathing patients or attending to dressings and carrying out treatment, they are *physically* exposed. Therefore the step towards exposing themselves *emotionally* is not great. Confidences are made and problems aired, which, perhaps like the hurting body-part, can be dealt with only behind screens or when there is total attention.

It is at these times that patients will come out with:

My husband and I never talk about dying.
I had never said this to anybody, but. . .
How do you think I am getting on?
That patient over there worries me. I've never seen anybody so ill.
What if I can't walk any more?

All these subtle questions can have a straightforward practical answer. But the setting in which they are asked probably means that this is not what they need. They need the small space of person-to-person contact and, in a way, demand that you, the nurse, 'expose' yourself too by your helping.

The situation may also be the other way round. There may be some patients who have never said anything remotely personal or which showed any self-awareness, and *you* feel that they have a problem that should be discussed. How do you go about it? This is far more delicate because you are imposing your values and standards on another person. All the communication skills you have are then needed. It is possible that, by showing your concern to them, patients may respond. It is possible that they may choose not you, but the least likely person in the team to confide in. What you cannot do is make somebody talk. You cannot 'counsel' someone; you can only help them to ask for counselling, if that is what they need. Brown (1988, p. 411) writes:

The comment of the mother of a 30-year-old man who died angry, in physical pain and mental torment, makes us stop and think. When one of the doctors explained how sad the team was, and felt that they had been able to help John so little, his mother said 'But he was an angry young man. He was a fighter all his life, and I'm glad you didn't change him'.

There are numerous practical problems that interfere with making the most of an opportunity: you talk with a patient and just then the telephone rings, your bleep goes, or you are called to an emergency. However much you try, you cannot really return to the patient and the subject easily. Or a patient may catch you just as you are going out of the door after a heavy day, when you have no more physical or emotional strength left. Or you go into the room of a very sick person whose hand lies on the bed begging to be held. Fear of what to say, or embarrassment, may make you pretend not to notice it, and instead busy yourself with all sorts of extras, like clearing out dead flowers.

Opportunities present themselves at every turn. Some you can deal with, some not. It may not matter so much when you *cannot* deal with them, for the patients will understand that. The difficulty is when you *won't* deal with them. You can't be giving all the time. When you can't, simply acknowledge your need. That in itself will be helpful.

Perhaps just as often you see an opportunity and you realize that there is simply no time because of too much administrative pressure. Who needs your skills more: the patient or the manager? By spending time with a patient you are neglecting your managerial duties. Your conscience may be torn between a real human need and a perhaps less urgent duty but one which ensures that your ward or unit can continue to function. Only you can make a decision. Your level of awareness, the amount of support you have for your work, and your values and job satisfaction will eventually guide you in your decisions.

Making a contract

A contract makes the difference between counselling and the use of counselling skills (British Association for Counselling, 1989).

A contract is a working agreement between helper and client, and can take many forms. Even just giving a time limit, or deciding to meet again, or asking for space is a form of contract.

Patient: I know you are busy, but have you got a minute?

Nurse: I've got ten minutes, is that enough?

Patient: I see you are just going home, but I've been trying to catch you all day.

Nurse: How urgent is the problem? You are right, I am on my way home.

Patient: Well, it won't go away, but it can wait until tomorrow.

Nurse: I will make a point of seeing you tomorrow morning.

Patient: Thank you, that will be fine.

Nurse: It seems to me that there is plenty more there to talk about.

Patient: I've had enough for one day now.

Nurse: Would you like me to come again tomorrow?

Patient: Not tomorrow, but Saturday. I won't have any visitors then.

Nurse: That's fine, I'm working late on Saturday. It's a deal.

Bayne et al. (1994, p. 27) say that a contract normally has two elements: 'one concerned with the purpose of counselling and your approach, the other with practical arrangements and conditions'. But these and other authors are all agreed that contracts have to be flexible and that many points can be covered. A contract could easily be seen as something imposed by a powerful expert on a weak and needy client. Helping is a 'collaborative venture' (Egan, 1994, p. 62) which includes rights and responsibilities for both parties. This may need to be made clear. Generally, an explicit contract with a client spells out how often they will meet, for how long, what it costs (if appropriate) and how and when payment should be made, what the conditions are for cancellation and whether the client is welcome to contact the counsellor between sessions.

Even when you are using counselling skills as part of your functional role, that is, of nursing, it may be good practice to inform the patient that you have these skills, that you are using them, and that you may be using a particular model. This can help the patient to know that there is some 'professionalism' present.

In mental health settings contracts play a large role, often as part of social skills training. People who are out of touch with social boundaries can gradually be reintroduced to living alongside other people by respecting such contracts. Nurses working in such settings will necessarily be trained in making contracts.

Whatever kind of contract you have established with a client, the important thing is that it is kept. If you have ten minutes to give to a person, give the ten minutes wholly, not thinking of all the other things you could be doing instead. If you say ten minutes, given ten, not eight or twenty minutes. If you do set time aside to talk with a patient, perhaps tell a colleague that you do not want to be disturbed.

Above all, if possible, never make assumptions: 'Oh, I know what my client wants anyway'. This time the client may want something different. The person who wants a 'word' with you may need many such words, and immediately; or this may simply be the only perceived way of asking you for something that may take just a sentence to answer. Check it out. Can it wait for your convenience or would it add to your client's pain and yours if you did not deal with it at once?

Transference and counter-transference

'Transference is the displacing of an emotion or attitude from one relationship to another' (Bayne et al, 1994, p. 154). There can be both positive and negative transference. Generally it means that feelings and emotions belonging properly to previous relationships are transferred on to a current relationship. Such feelings are inappropriate, intense, ambivalent and inconsistent (Stewart, 1992). Peck (1993, p. 238) calls it 'the outdated map'.

The concept of transference is particularly associated with Freud, who used the concept to discover more about the emotional states and early life of his patients. Counselling is less geared to calling up unconscious material deliberately, so that transference is less of a specific tool in this type of helping. Nevertheless, transference is very often present.

Patients in hospital sometimes behave as if they were in love with nurses when, in fact, they invest in the nurse the love which they feel for their mother. Relatives may be afraid to ask doctors for their opinion and may treat doctors with the deference which might have been appropriate for their own fathers. Parents often transfer to their children's teacher the mixture of fear and respect they formerly had for their own headmaster. Nurses may find that their attitude towards the sister or nursing officer is irrational and represents a transference of feelings from their own family experience. (Altschul and Sinclair, 1981, p. 130)

Some of these feelings are misplaced and irrational, but because of their very existence they are important and may throw light on other feelings or behaviours. Clients use us (and we use others) to act out relationships with other significant people in their (or our) lives.

Miller (1981) says that transference is

essentially a defence mechanism, designed to protect ourselves and preserve our security. Knowing ourselves may be threatening, and the more threatening it is, the more likely a person is to project.

A transference, or projection, is always about a feeling, usually an unfinished feeling from the past, and is often not related clearly to what is going on now. However, if such feelings can be faced and used, they can become integral parts of the helping process and lead the patient or client to own the past and the present with a view to being a more whole and 'potent' person in the future.

Transference means that a patient projects a feeling on to you; in counter-transference you then project back to the client your own unacknowledged feelings. If you let yourself act in the role in which you are cast by the client, then you counter-transfer. According to Stewart (1992, p. 279), transference is present in most intimate relationships, it is natural, and it is reduced with accurate empathy.

Involvement

The fear of getting involved with patients is rather pernicious. It is a fear of not being able to stand back from a situation and then being swept along into areas of patients' lives that may encroach too closely on one's own. Such fears can be more destructive than the actual 'getting involved' itself.

I have argued in this book that to help others emotionally, you need to deal with their feelings. It is the feelings that have priority in helping. Feelings need empathy to be understood, experienced and managed. Without empathy, feelings run away with us, overpower and frighten us. With empathy, feelings become our friends and helpers. Now empathy is a way of being: being with people and their feelings. It is also a way of being with ourselves and our feelings. This means that we are *already* 'involved'. This means that we should be involved appropriately. This demands first of all an awareness: of what is going on; of pitfalls and blind spots; of fears and short-comings. But, just as individual clients are unable to extricate themselves from a difficult situation, so we, the helpers, also need support, probably in the form of supervision.

Simply to say 'don't get involved' does not help. If you say this to a colleague it may come from your own fear of getting close to people, or from a bad experience. Your colleague may have no difficulty with getting close. If it is said to you, perhaps you should question the assumptions that have led to the remark being made. Everyone understands 'involvement' differently. With empathy you can go down into the ditch and be with the other person, knowing that you still have one foot on firm ground. Empathy can then mean that you hear the story the other has to tell, be all there, and also able to introduce new and different perspectives and thus enable and empower the person to go on his or her own way again.

If you do feel involved or caught in a trap – which can always happen – then the best thing to do is to discuss it with a colleague, supervisor or other trusted person. Panic reactions like asking to be moved to a different area of work may not be the best solution as this may only increase the sense of hurt and failure. Dealing with a problem is better for clients; it is also better for nurses.

Involvement usually points to a counter-transference situation: you are projecting on to another person some unfinished relationship business from the past. Counter-transference can be a strong and unrecognized trap and, being a trap, there is no way out of it alone. But with the companionship of empathy it can be seen again for what it is, acknowledged, and changed.

Dependence on clients

Transference and counter-transference are not the same as the helper's need to be needed.

Helpers do not only have needs to be helped; they have deep needs to be needed. There is nothing wrong in that. It becomes dangerous only when this need is misused, either by yourself or by others.

You were probably asked at your original interview why you wanted to go into nursing and you probably answered that you wanted to help people. If you were further asked why you wanted to help people, you might have said that you wanted to care for people less fortunate than you or less well than you.

When you are helping clients to deal with important aspects of their lives, you are likely to ask them for the (or a) meaning in their lives. This may uncover a number of unknown elements.

As helpers we need to be willing to be challenged, and therefore be willing to examine the meaning or purpose of our own life at critical moments. We can only ask others what we can also ask of ourselves. We can only teach others what we also know ourselves. In a way, we can only do to others what we also do to ourselves. We love others only when we love ourselves. We are nurses to others only when we know how to be nurses to ourselves. We hurt others only because we also hurt ourselves. We need others only because we are needy in ourselves.

Human nature is such that we *do* need each other for living. But to *use* others to boost ourselves is unhelpful for both parties; in that case, neither side can grow. When you come to the awareness, and act on it, that you walk side by side on the road of life, not carried on each other's backs, then you set each other free.

When you acknowledge your needs, they become tools for you to work with, rather than luggage that you demand others to carry for you. When you allow yourself to acknowledge your needs, you become free to help. Then your needs will be met by all those you help; but that is incidental. It does not happen if you ask your clients to fulfil your needs, thus keeping them dependent on you.

This chapter has highlighted once again the various and often hidden agendas that each person has. As a helper you have just as many as your clients have. All of these issues are not either right or wrong. They simply *are*. The way you *are* with them is what matters.

One of the comments about counselling sometimes made by teachers and tutors is that it is impossible to know what is 'their' and what is 'your' (my) business. Looking at this issue in the light of awareness, and perhaps transference and counter-transference, and how they are set up and maintained, may help to make the distinction and lessen the burden or confusion.

CHAPTER THIRTEEN

Specific situations

It is impossible to say that one type of nurse or another is more vulnerable or that this situation or that is more difficult. Any situation or problem can be easy or difficult, depending on any number of factors. What is easy for one person is difficult for another. The difference lies in the experience of the practitioner. Helping and counselling are not fixes, but interactions between people, some of whom are more vulnerable than others some of the time.

Sometimes you will be faced with completely unexpected situations or remarks, and you are inevitably surprised. Nursing will have taught you a certain unshockability. Together with a non-judgemental attitude and perhaps an ability to see the funny side of things occasionally will be vital if you want to use your counselling skills.

Clients with learning disabilities

People with learning disabilities are usually well cared for by specialist nurses. While forty years ago most of them died before they reached their teens, today most live beyond the age of 40 (Smith, 1994). They are therefore likely to be admitted to acute settings for care at some time in their lives. The problems then are not just to do with the presenting illness.

Often through long years of earlier institutionalization, people with learning disabilities are used to having decisions made for them, even having a sentence finished for them. Taking responsibility for themselves is therefore something that they may neither understand nor be willing to do.

The points in life when people with learning disabilities need counselling are often to do with major decisions in their lives, such as moving from an institution to a home, or into the community. It may be very difficult for people with a learning disability to understand what this involves for them, or what they are expected to do. Riley (1983) found that most of her difficulties were 'pitching what you say at the right level so that you are both talking about the same thing'. Some things have to be stated very simply, and be repeated often. It may also be necessary to bear in mind that some disabled people have unusual facial expressions, so it may be difficult to gauge whether what has been said has been really understood, and whether the response will be as expected. There may be no outward sign of change in mood, and that may be difficult for the counsellor.

The difficulty that some clients have in expressing feelings does not mean that they do not have any. Helping people with learning disabilities to express their feelings may help them to bring meaning and wholeness into their lives, although perhaps not as quickly as for other people. Using counselling skills correctly is therefore even more important for this group of people, and perhaps even more rewarding in the end.

Counselling children

Young children have a different understanding and experience of the world from adults. Counselling in adult terms is therefore not relevant to small children. What matters is that they are heard and responded to at the appropriate level and in the appropriate manner.

It should be realized that very ill children often have an intuitive knowledge about death and dying. Explanations should be given in simple words and metaphors which they can understand, such as making comparisons with pets who have died.

More taxing for nurses is the help that parents need. It is they who bear a heavy burden with sick children. Despite what they may think, their children are often very astute at realizing when parents are worried or fearful. When the parents feel at ease, the child becomes at ease. Helping and counselling the parents may therefore be the priority.

Siblings tend to be the forgotten party in these situations. The parents have to care for the sick child, and siblings are left to cope. Although they may not have much contact with hospital nursing staff, the situation in the community is quite different. Here, a nurse may get to know the family situation well and find it particularly appropriate to consider the family as a whole when offering help. It may also be possible for community nurses to make a special point to ask after the welfare of the siblings, and even address them themselves to hear their own stories.

The 'problem' patient

There will always be people with whom you have difficulty developing a fruitful relationship. You try to help, but they refuse help. You try to cajole, and they don't want to know. You try to humour them, and they think you don't take them seriously.

Perhaps the most difficult patients are those who ask for your help but reject it. They do this to everybody else: each nurse will hear the story, and it is normally a long one. Day after day they drain you of your energy. What is more, having done the round of all the possible people, they are then in a position to play one person off against another. 'Do you know what the physio suggested? She said I should lose weight! What an effrontery!' Because of a respect for confidentiality, you are caught in a web of intrigue. The patient wants help, but is not able to use the help offered.

Such patients are themselves caught in a world of fantasy and make-believe. They think that they are victims and need to be rescued. And nurses, like most health care workers, have a strong sense of rescuing, and they are seduced.

The story of the person in the ditch (see Chapter 6) shows quite clearly that he was not rescued, but helped to stand on his own feet, and so could walk away from the spot under his own steam. People who take on the role of victim have been hurt somewhere in life, but that behaviour is now not relevant any more and should if possible be challenged. Moreover, what they present as a problem is unlikely to be the real problem, which they cannot talk about because, if they did, they would expose a side of themselves that is weak, helpless and quite inadequate. So they play the game of deception.

Patient: Nurse, will you help me sort this out?
Nurse: I'll try.
Patient: I spoke to Nurse J yesterday, but she was so rude that I don't want to speak to her any more.

The trap here is to be shocked by Nurse J's remark and so get away from the problem.

Nurse: How can I help you?
Patient: Well, you said I could go home next week, but you see I can't use that arm at all well, and how can I look after myself with one useless arm and the other not strong enough?
Nurse: We've talked about that several times already and there all sorts of possibilities.
Patient: But you don't understand! I simply have no-one to help me.

Another trap: you don't understand me. The nurse is made to feel that she is no good, or should defend herself.

Nurse: I'm beginning to feel that you are afraid of something at home. You've lived alone so long.

Patient: You nurses are all the same. You never believe what anybody says and read things into situations which you don't know anything about.

The patient becomes defensive. This probably proves that the nurse is on to something 'real'.

Nurse: Are you afraid of something at home?
Patient: Of course not, what makes you think that?
Nurse: I just thought I could detect a note of fear in your voice.
Patient: I'm all right.
Nurse: I just have a hunch that something is not all right.
Patient: I don't have a problem at home.
Nurse: Is the problem somewhere else?
Patient: You are persistent, aren't you?

This may mean: leave me alone. Or it may mean: you are right, go on.

Nurse: I am, but tell me if I'm not right.
Patient: Well. . .
Nurse: What is it, can you tell me?
Patient: It's a long story, but I just hate that flat.
Nurse: Go on.

This story (the patient eventually revealed that she hated her flat because her husband had died there; she felt that she had killed him and the memory constantly haunted her) shows that by not giving in to the many traps laid, but by (1) concentrating on the patient and her feelings, and (2) following her intuition, the nurse got to a point where something could be 'moved'. The patient's own defence mechanism kept her locked into a situation that was increasingly unbearable and unproductive, not to mention the undesirability of keeping her in care and dependent when she could be independent. In this case the nurse referred the patient to a social worker who helped her with her long-term emotional problem as well as with housing.

Relatives

Sometimes the problem is not the patient, but the family. At the bedside of the patient are acted out all manner of family dynamics which perhaps were never dealt with before.

Those who were formerly independent and dominant will have become dependent, and vice versa. The role of carer and cared-for will have been reversed. It is easy to underestimate the immense process of adjustment involved in this change. Children find it difficult to come to terms with the responsibilities involved, and parents find it difficult to relinquish them. (Scrutton, 1989, p. 91)

This means that situations of 'Don't tell him, he couldn't cope' or 'I'm the spokesperson for the family' arise and power games begin to be played out. As the nurse, you are in the middle, trying to keep the parties either together or apart.

It is an understatement to say that this is not easy. As a nurse you have your own feelings and values to consider, and your own, the patient's and the family's integrity to maintain.

Like the patient, the family may accept or reject your help. Like the patient, you can only offer help but not make them take it. You cannot 'counsel' them if they are not willing to be helped. But your empathic approach may be perceived as genuinely caring, and will be appreciated as such.

Depending on how long the patient remains in your care, you may be able to loosen some knots that may be preventing free-flowing relationships. You may be able to present a different point of view from the one held by the family and so bring in a different perspective that might be acceptable. You may be able to use your position in the middle as a real go-between and help to heal old rifts. You may be able to place anger and resentments where they properly belong (in the past) by helping both sides to see what they are doing to each other.

Helping and counselling members of the family is the same as helping and counselling patients. The only thing to keep in mind, if you are helping both sides, is that their respective confidences have to be kept separate unless you have permission from one side or the other to pass on anything relevant.

Families often rely on nurses as much as the patients themselves do, and it can be rewarding to leave a whole family unit in a better state than when it first came into your care.

Dying and death

The care of dying people has received a great deal of attention in recent years, and more and more nurses, not only those in hospices, feel increasingly comfortable with it. Nevertheless, most nurses still fear the outright question, 'Am I dying?', although experience shows that it is seldom asked in this way but more likely as:

Do you think I'm really getting better?
I know it will soon be my turn.
It's a funny thing, dying. I can understand now why people will try
every treatment they can get.

Kübler-Ross (1969) was one of the first people who classified
the process of dying into stages. Since then, the subject has
been much written about and from every conceivable angle.
The essential elements of the process are: denial, anger, fear
and resolution. It is important to realize that here, too, the
stages can be muddled up, and a patient who one day is angry,
may the next day be accepting the situation, and the third day
be paralysed with fear. Brown (1988, p. 415) lists the principles
of help and support given to people who are dying as: (1) never
tell a lie; (2) never take away all hope; (3) listen well.

Brown gives a good example of how these principles have
been put into action (p. 413).

Mrs Todd was a 46-year-old patient with a glioma. One new develop-
ment on the day before the following conversation was the onset of
marked weakness in her right leg. The nurse had taken Mrs Todd her
night-time medication, and had listened while Mrs Todd told her some
of the day's events, and of her husband's and children's visits that
evening. As the nurse turned to go, Mrs Todd called her back.

Patient: 'Nurse!'
The nurse turned and took the few steps back toward the bed.
Patient: 'Do you think I might die suddenly in the night?'
           A categoric 'No' would certainly have been unhelpful and
           possibly untrue. Mrs Todd could have a haemorrhage into
           the tumour, or indeed, she could have a heart attack. Pati-
           ents with cancer are not immune from these, but neither
           was there a high degree of likelihood, and to have men-
           tioned them would have served no useful purpose.
Nurse: 'I think that is highly unlikely, Mrs Todd.'
           The temptation was to hurry back to the medicine trolley,
           but there were likely to be more worries behind Mrs Todd's
           question. She would probably go on only if she felt the nurse
           had time. This was communicated much more clearly non-
           verbally than it could have been verbally. Staying, sitting,
           and sharing concerned attention, helped Mrs Todd to go
           on to ask about another patient in the ward.
Patient: 'But Mrs Green over there has been getting up much less*
           lately, and today she's been in bed all day, and has
           hardly stirred.'

Nurse: 'Yes, she has been getting gradually more tired and sleepy over the past few days.'

Patient: 'Do you think that will happen to me?'

Nurse: 'Yes, I think it probably will when the time comes, though not just yet.'

Patient: 'What do the nurses do when they pull the curtains round her bed every so often?'

Nurse: 'Well the nurses move Mrs Green's position so that she does not become sore. If you look next time the nurses have been to her, you'll find she is facing the opposite way. They also moisten her mouth to keep it comfortable, now that she cannot drink.'

Patient: 'And her husband? He has been sitting there all day – my husband won't be able to do that. He can't bear being here, and doesn't stay very long. What will the nurses think of him?'

Nurse: 'It is important for relatives to do what feels right and comfortable for them. We will try to help him to do that. His way may be different, but not better or worse.'

Patient: 'And that bag – will I have one of those? Now my leg is weaker, I have to have a commode by the bed, but what if I can't make it out of bed? I couldn't bear to make a mess.'

Nurse: 'Yes, if that should happen we will be able to use a catheter to drain the urine as we have with Mrs Green.'

Patient: 'I have been so worried today, not knowing what was happening to Mrs Green; and yet she seems comfortable and peaceful, and still cared for. But it helps to know what's happening. Thank you. You must get on now, and I'll get to sleep.'

The next morning, Mrs Todd told one of the doctors that, since she had been ill, she had wondered what dying would be like. It had helped to talk about what was happening to Mrs Green.

Nurses often feel that they should answer a straight 'Am I dying?' with a straight 'yes' or 'no'. They say that *they* would like to know if they asked that question. One way of looking at this dilemma is with the help of the Four Questions (see Chapter 5).

1. *What is happening?* The client will have some reason for asking that question. He/she may not be feeling well; certain investigations will have aroused suspicion; some remarks dropped were perhaps not very clear. The client will therefore have reached some sort of conclusion

already. In all this there will probably also be a great deal of fear, anger, guilt and any number of other possible emotions.

A straight, simple question is therefore like a digest of all these factors. To give a simple answer may be like putting a match to a can of petrol and causing an explosion. Asking 'What is happening?' may not only avoid an emotional explosion, but perhaps enable a cleansing fire to burn old and unhealthy parts of the personality.

Instead of saying 'yes', asking 'What is happening?' ('What makes you ask me?'; 'What do you yourself believe to be the case?' etc) gives not only space to the helper, but also enables clients to express themselves more and perhaps disclose any fears and other circumstances that may have led to the question in the first place. Clients can benefit from hearing themselves tell their stories, and helpers gain valuable insights.

2. *What is the meaning of it?* Clients will probably not be as concerned with their actual death as with what this suffering, illness, physical and emotional pain is all about. Someone concerned with finding meaning or significance is not concerned with details.

Helping clients to voice their fears and pains may lead them naturally and by themselves to see the meaning of them. The 'problem', that is, the question of whether the client is dying, may then solve itself. This is not a cop-out for helpers so that they do not have to answer, but all of us know that when we have reached our own conclusions, we are more satisfied. We do not give others their meaning, but we help them to discover the meaning that is there for them. Helpers may then simply need to confirm what clients and patients have known anyway.

3. *What is your goal?* Why did the client ask the question? Probably not because of any concern at this moment about the minutiae of dying, but to make sense of what is ahead.

The concern should therefore be to help such people come to their own conclusions and in their own time. What do they understand by dying? What do they expect death to be like? What would they like to happen about dying, and about death itself?

It may be paradoxical to think of death as a goal. Yet, most people have some idea of how and where they would like to die. There are many practical aspects to death, and when clients can be helped to be in charge of their life, then dying is not decline, but growth, and death itself not just an inevitable end, but something with which they can cooperate.

4. *How are you going to do it?* When patients have the emotional wherewithal to cope with dying, then, like Mrs Todd, they can begin to think of the practicalities of dying and take the necessary steps. They may suddenly find the energy to do this. But there will also be some clients who give up and turn to the wall, not wanting to know anything more. Respecting this is just as important as is helping those who have a new agenda.

'Never telling a lie' does not mean that you should always tell 'the truth'. What is truth to you may not be truth to the client. The client's truth comes out of the experience of living with disease and illness. Your truth may come out of the case-notes and pathology reports; these truths are not necessarily the same. This shows most clearly why it is so important to respond to the *person*, not the problem.

Bereavement

Grieving after death is different only in context from grieving before death. Both aspects mourn someone or something lost. The dying person mourns a personal loss of life, health and all that is important then. The bereaved person mourns the loss of the beloved one's life. The stages of both processes are remarkably similar.

An illness often brings back a multitude of memories, and losses are the strongest memories. Many people are grieving for people and things lost ten, twenty, fifty years earlier. It may not be evident at once that that is the problem, but as soon as you touch on the meaning of a present crisis, the possibility of unfinished grief is very real.

Clients may grieve over events and situations which may not always be obvious, such as the loss of a house, or an abortion. Nurses and helpers generally need to be aware that clients may not have given enough attention to particular memories.

The traumas surrounding stillbirth and perinatal death have been recognized more readily recently. Self-help groups and advice centres exist for women and families with this type of bereavement. But still the effects may last for many years and be devastating.

Women who have had abortions may never receive any kind of help. The decision to have an abortion is often a quick one, taken when the person is under pressure. An abortion can literally be done in the lunch-break and nobody need know about it. It may only be years later that the effects are felt, when the person may be feeling too shy, guilty, or helpless to talk about it. A non-judgemental attitude could then be the key to unloading a great deal of grief and freeing the person to live more satisfyingly again.

The death of a pet animal is more often considered to be traumatic for children, but adults too, and especially older people, may feel seriously bereaved when a dog or cat dies. Often their whole life revolves around an animal, which then becomes the 'significant other', having been invested with human properties. If such a pet is lost it may be more devastating than if a close person died. The effects should never be belittled or treated lightly.

A particularly valuable text in the area of bereavement is Worden's (1994) *Grief Counselling and Grief Therapy*, which sheds much light on many situations and problems encountered by health care personnel.

Spiritual aspects

Coming face to face with one's own mortality may raise questions about spiritual and religious matters. For many patients, and nurses, this is not something with which they are familiar.

When you are listening to a person, you will be hearing what a person is about. You may be able to point to something spiritual which the person might not have recognized. Or the patient may talk to you about God, and that is not an easy subject for you. The genuineness, warmth and empathy always required in counselling are needed here too, where often our own bias and needs are obvious.

Referral

One of the things most people need to learn early on is that they have limits. You can help some people, but not others. You can do so much, but not everything. You will sooner or later come across situations that are beyond your skills. But at least you have uncovered the problem.

Any referral should be made only in the client's best interest. Those clients who have trusted you with parts of themselves and their lives may find it difficult to confide in someone else. This should be borne in mind. You should therefore be quite sure why you intend to suggest a referral. The most likely reason is that the problem presented is clearly the province of somebody else, such as a social worker, chaplain or psychiatrist. When you have good reason, you should seek specialist help where applicable. If this is not the best way forward, you may need to consider dealing with the situation yourself, perhaps with the express help of a supervisor.

When referral is the appropriate way forward in a counselling situation, this should be discussed with the client, whose consent to it is necessary. But even when someone else may do most of the counselling, you may still need to be around with care and concern, and not cut the client off completely. A referral may not be available straight away, and so you may need to help the person not only to accept other help, but to make the transition, and to cover the period between the two helpers.

Nurse (1980) suggests that we should help clients to make their own application for referral. When you can lead people, through counselling, to manage their own problems, including where to go for specialist help, then the helping process has come full circle. One final aspect of referral is that it

must not be seen as failure on the counsellor's part. On the contrary, it is an ingredient of the whole process of helping, and skill is needed to identify when this is the most appropriate step to take. (Nurse, 1980, p. 90)

If you have discovered the problem in the first place, then you have done the most important part of the work.

Difficult situations are only one aspect of work; they are only that part of it which gives you cause for concern. The other aspects are all the situations that give you joy and job satisfaction, and make you feel good. But, as always, for wholeness in life, both are needed, both challenge us to greater things.

CHAPTER FOURTEEN

Ethical issues

....

This book is written specifically for nurses who use counselling skills as part of their role as nurses. This may include specific counselling opportunities, but always within the wider framework of nursing. The ethical components are therefore somewhat different from those that apply to people who call themselves counsellors by profession.

Some basic concepts of ethics

Ethics is not only the study of right and wrong. It also asks *why* right and wrong, and right and wrong in relation to what?

Chambers Dictionary (1993) describes ethics as 'the science of morals, that branch of philosophy which is concerned with human character and conduct' and 'a system of morals or rules of behaviour'. Inevitably, there is not just one such set of rules or one view of how humans should behave. If there were, there would be no more free will, and that has often been regarded as the starting point of ethics as a study and of ethical behaviour.

There are two broad strands in ethics. The first is *deontology* (the science of duty or 'ought'), also referred to as non-consequentialism. It focuses on rights, duties and principles, and is particularly concerned with establishing codes of ethics. The other strand is *teleology* (the science of final causes), also known as consequentialism or utilitarianism. This area focuses on the actions that produce the greatest good. Much of medical ethics, and indeed the establishment of the National Health Service, rests on this theory.

Despite differences, both orientations are accepted by philosophers as worthy of serious consideration. Both strive to be logical and consistent, and often come to similar decisions in morally similar situations.

Any broad theory has to be made accessible and functional. A series of principles is therefore often established. By focusing on such principles it is hoped that ethical problems and dilemmas can be solved. At least, this has been the reasoning behind much teaching on ethics.

In recent years the pendulum has begun to swing away from theories and principles. Practitioners have been disappointed with theories and found them limiting and immobile in practice, where most problems are dealt with on a basis of common sense and without the use of theories with obscure names and principles which demand mental gymnastics. The argument now is that people are well enough equipped with a sense of morality anyway and do and need to rely on their personal capacity to reason. This may be a reaction to the sudden growth of all things ethical and may therefore be useful. Perhaps when the pendulum comes to rest again somewhere, we may find that common sense *and* principles, natural morality *and* theories need to be used in critical situations. For this reason a set of principles is briefly described here.

Thiroux (1980) writes about five principles that apply generally. Many nurses will be familiar with the writings of Beauchamp and Childress (1989). As these authors write specifically for medicine, the principles they advocate are not always equally valid for nursing and it may therefore be better to use a more general system to cover the combined areas of nursing, counselling and ethics here. Thiroux (1980) considers the principles of the value of life, goodness or rightness, justice or fairness, truth-telling or honesty, and individual freedom.

The principle of the value of life

Thiroux sums up this principle with the simple phrase: 'Human beings should revere life and accept death' (p. 124). Most of the world's moral systems have some prohibition on killing. People who value (human) life as good in itself will want to be sure that they are not killed, and they will not kill others. But principles can at best be near-absolutes, not absolutes, and this principle is infringed in cases of abortion, euthanasia, killing in self-defence, war, capital punishment and suicide.

The principle is also infringed in many less dramatic ways. Revering life does not only mean biological life, but 'living' in its widest sense. This means respecting our own and other people's ways of being, thinking and behaving. This shows up obvious wrong-doing (and the law has to deal with this), but the demarcation line between right and wrong is not necessarily clear and is the constant theme of ethics. Many of the issues discussed in this book from a counselling point of view also apply from an ethical viewpoint.

Nurses will meet this principle in matters of care at every turn: abortion, care of the dying, decisions regarding resuscitation, the way in which people are treated, and much more. The way in which you care for others depends largely on how you value life and living.

The principle of goodness or rightness

Ethics is the study of good and right: 'good' human beings should attempt to perform 'right' actions. But what or who is a good person, and in relation to what is that person good? Who establishes good, and who judges it?

To live in a harmonious world, Thiroux (1980) maintains, human beings should attempt to do three things:

1, promote goodness over badness; 2, cause no harm or badness; and 3, prevent badness or harm.

The basic guidelines for this behaviour are the professional codes. The *Code of Professional Conduct for the Nurse, Midwife and Health Visitor* (United Kingdom Central Council, 1992), the *Code of Ethics and Practice for Counsellors* (British Association for Counselling, 1993) and the *Code of Ethics and Practice for Counselling Skills* (British Association for Counselling, 1989) are the documents mainly relevant here. By dealing with issues of responsibility, integrity, competence and confidentiality, both personally and professionally, such codes lay down parameters within which the person should function so that both the individual professional and the profession, the individual client and society at large benefit, and good is actively promoted and bad or harm prevented.

The principle of justice and fairness

This is a principle that is increasingly important and increasingly more difficult to keep. Essentially it means that all citizens have the same rights and that there should be no discrimination. The recent growth in charters of every kind promotes this idea. But in practice everyone knows that it does not work like that and that some people are 'more equal than others'.

All nurses know how difficult it is to make just decisions and how demoralizing it is when patients and clients do not get what they should by right. Many counselling situations will be concerned with the issues of justice. How is it possible to do no harm when there are not enough resources to go round everybody? The decision to speak out against injustice is never taken lightly, and the values or virtues of personal courage, loyalty and integrity must play a large part.

The principle of truth telling or honesty

Our whole moral system rests on telling the truth. Unless we are sure to be given truthful information, life itself would be untenable. Even when we buy a packet of tea we need to be sure that there is tea in it, and not something else. Equally, you need to pay with honest (real) money, not counterfeit.

In medicine, 'the patient has a *legal right* (author's italics) to expect his medical adviser to take all proper steps to elucidate the truth about his condition' (Duncan et al, 1981). This is the doctor's duty. The difficulty arises because truth telling cannot be made a legal *duty* but is an ethical imperative.

This principle is infringed by any untruth, white lie, insincerity or misrepresentation. But against this must be put the fact that our relationships are a complicated web of being with people in which we reveal only certain parts of ourselves to others. Human vulnerability is nowhere so obvious as in personal and business relationships. Perhaps most counselling interventions concern relationships and their ramifications. It is not a question of 'the truth, the whole truth and nothing but the truth' under this heading; it is much more a question of what 'the truth' means to someone, and how much that person is prepared to have and to live.

The principle of individual freedom

Morality cannot exist if human beings are not to some extent free to make moral choices and decisions. Human beings are unique and individual, and therefore have the opportunity to express themselves individually, in and through their lives, and particularly in relationships with other individual human beings. They would have neither individuality nor freedom if the ethical principles were absolutes. But neither freedom itself, nor even moral freedom, is absolute.

As free individuals, we are also autonomous. But autonomy does not mean unconditional freedom. Benjamin and Curtis (1986, p. 23) say that

Ethical autonomy involves thinking for *oneself, not* of *oneself or* by *oneself. Thinking* for *oneself is usually more successful if it includes*

at least some thinking with *others. One may perfectly well think* for *oneself and still think* about *and* with *others.*

This principle stresses equality: the equality of people in moral matters. The Golden Rule, 'Do unto others as you would be done by', stresses this point of equality in moral matters. Despite the fact that we are not all social, religious or economic equals, we are all morally equal as persons. The first four principles, of the value of life, goodness, justice and honesty, give us a moral framework, and within them we need to be free to express our individuality, our freedom, and our equality.

This principle is particularly relevant in helping and counselling. As a helper you have the freedom to give or withhold help, when and to whom you give it. Your choice should therefore be a moral one.

You are in a position of influence. Your clients, by the very fact of being clients, are vulnerable. How you use your influence is therefore crucial.

Without thinking about it, and without perhaps realizing it, you are constantly making ethical decisions. This should not be a cause for alarm but should lead you to constantly greater awareness and the general commitment to your own personal and professional growth. As you review your techniques of helping, so you review your values, and your ethical principles in and of helping.

Personal values and convictions

Underlying any ethical reasoning and caring are the values that we hold and by which we live. Some of these may be quite unconscious; some may have been instilled by our parents and teachers and are therefore more theirs than ours; and some may have been consciously chosen for particular reasons. Caring is one such value.

By caring you respond to something that matters. Your caring matters, and the 'other' that you respond to matters. The way in which you respond to people, events and objects expresses your values. An affective response to someone or something is not simply emotivism. 'It is an intentional response, deliberate, meaningful and rational' (Roach, 1992, p. 64).

That response stems out of a person's conscience. 'Conscience grows out of experience, out of a process of valuing self and others. Conscience is the call of care and manifests itself as care' (Roach, 1992, p. 64). Conscience is more than a censor of morals; it is the basis and the direction of that which we live by: our values and convictions.

When people have reached a 'moment of truth' which may bring them to ask for help, this is likely to be a moment when their values are suddenly questioned or overturned. What counted until now simply does not count any more. A process of discovery of new values, new meanings and new goals has to start. That is often not possible on one's own.

As a helper you are not in such a crisis. Your own values and way of being may therefore act as a guideline to help other individuals to find their own way. However, somewhere, some time in the past, you will also have had your 'moment of truth', when you were tested, buffeted and had to grope for new light. This may be the basis for the humility that helpers need, in order to 'identify' with their clients. It may also be your strength, because you have come through it and can use that fact as an encouragement to your client, by sharing some of your experience.

The value of any experience lies in its meaning. The values and convictions you hold are expressions of the meanings in your life. When these are used in the service of others then you are not only a competent counsellor, you are also an ethical helper. The following headings look more specifically at the ethical components of helping and counselling within nursing.

Competence

It has been said that when learning a new subject we move from

unconscious incompetence to
conscious incompetence to
conscious competence to
unconscious competence.

Those who do not know about a particular subject are not going to teach others about it and are therefore harmless. But those who believe that they do know a subject, such as counselling, when in fact they do not, are downright dangerous. Helping other people is a serious matter and can be potentially disastrous. Yet this does not mean that only fully qualified people can help others. On the contrary, learning about counselling and learning how to do it has to be done 'live'. Nurses who are taking courses in counselling and counselling skills will be supervised and helped and will have constant reminders about awareness. They will also be taught the essentials of self-monitoring their practice.

Those nurses who have had no training and who have no supervision run the greatest risks of being ineffective or unconsciously incompetent.

There is at present no one authority to monitor competence in either counselling or the use of counselling skills. In September 1994 the British Association for Counselling 'set up a method and facility within its structure to allow for the development of a United Kingdom Register of Counsellors (UKRC). It is intended that the structure for the Register will be in place early in 1996 and develop from that date' (British Association for Counselling, 1994b).

The problem is not just official recognition of competence, but, as always, how to deal with dangerous and incompetent practitioners. At present, any nurse who either counsels or uses counselling skills and who is deemed unsafe or incompetent in that area would automatically be judged by the United Kingdom Central Council (UKCC) as the primary professional regulator. Colleagues and clients who might make an official complaint would need to have proof of either incompetence or unprofessional conduct, and this could be very difficult to substantiate in the present circumstances.

Standards of care

While there is no agreed criterion of what is offered by helping and counselling, it is difficult to set standards that should be achieved. Even then, how is it possible to measure the value of empathy, or the number of tears shed (Charnock, 1985) by clients, or the quality of 'being with' another person? In the increasingly money-oriented and economy-driven health service, giving human care has more and more of a premium attached. Depending on your values, you either go along with the trends, fight them, or try to steer clear of them. Your stance may change depending on certain circumstances.

The common foundation programmes of Project 2000 courses feature such subjects as respect and dignity, partnership in caring, communication skills and ethics. As always, the credibility gap between theory and practice may turn out to be quite large when the nurses go to the communities and wards and there find the driving force to be value for money, not human well-being and dignity.

The UKCC Code of Professional Conduct (UKCC, 1992) says that 'as a registered nurse, midwife or health visitor, you are personally accountable for your practice and, in the exercise of your professional accountability, must: act always in such a manner as to promote and safeguard the interests and well-being of patients and clients'. The word 'must' is uncompromising, but what 'promoting' and 'safeguarding' stands for is less precise. The profession demands of its workers that they maintain certain levels or standards of care, but how they are maintained is the personal duty of each professional. In the area of helping and counselling this may sometimes have to be done by challenging concepts and ideals. When you believe that human values are as important as those of the money market, then you may sometimes have to say so very clearly. This is never easy in itself; it is even more difficult when your livelihood may thereby be put into question.

Responsibility

Most of our actions are responses to actions towards us. One way of expressing our humanity is by *responding* rather than just reacting. In the responses we make there will have been a choice. We have the ability to respond, which leads us to responsibility.

Most of the time there is a responsibility *to* something or someone. In terms of ethics, this responsibility is to

oneself
clients
colleagues
employers
profession
society

in that order, although this changes in certain circumstances.

The responsibility to oneself first of all is crucial. Unless we know why we are acting in a certain way, we are not acting ethically.

When you are helping clients or patients you do it from a sense of care-giving, duty, altruism or other motive. The basis from which you act is first of all a personal one: you give of yourself. If you are asked to give of yourself in a situation in which you are not at ease, such as when you are coerced, then you cannot truly give of yourself. Or what you give is less than good enough. There is conflict and your integrity is compromised.

Many nurses do find themselves in this predicament. They are asked to care in situations in which they are not free to respond ethically, that is, responsibly. This may be with clients and patients, but is more often seen to be through pressure from management or more senior colleagues. When the way to respond personally is impossible, conflict arises.

The responsibility to clients is often not clear. 'Duty of care' is something that is perhaps more often used as a stick than as a carrot, and in ways that are not clearly spelled out. In the area of counselling this is even more difficult to define. It is impossible to ask a person to give counselling help, but when it is not given – and when it could and should have been given – then there is a clear lack of responsibility.

The responsibility to colleagues in terms of counselling is perhaps made more difficult by the UKCC Code of Professional Conduct (1992) which states in Clause 13, that 'in the exercise of your professional accountability, (you) must: report to an appropriate person or authority where it appears that the health or safety of colleagues is at risk, as such circumstances may compromise standards of practice and care'. This clause does appear to be a licence to snoop rather than help effectively. Where helping has been attempted and failed, then it should indeed be made known, but ideally in such a way that the persons concerned are involved in ways that are as healthy and 'right' as possible.

What is done to and with one person is inevitably done to and with society. The ripples of any kind of interaction are wide and influence many people. The reputation of a ward, hospital or district does not depend on an anonymous collective, but on each individual – however embarrassing that may sometimes be.

Accountability

Responsibility leads to accountability. When helping clients by using counselling skills, there are the same spheres of accountability as there are for responsibility, except the first (self). The most authentic accountability is always to the clients, but in the way that help is given, colleagues, employers, the profession and society all have a right to demand accountability too. In practice this may be difficult. Employers do, however, often ask for breakdowns of how time is spent, and may question whether a person's use of time for counselling activities is justified or not. From time spent with clients alone it is not yet possible to say whether this is also quality time spent.

One of the skills that helpers and clients need to acquire is self-monitoring. Clearly, helpers and counsellors do not want to disclose confidential material when they are asked to account for their practice; therefore it is important to be sure what is required to be accounted for, when, to whom, and why.

Marks-Maran (1993, p. 124) distinguishes between legal, managerial, professional and moral accountability. When these categories are applied to the use of counselling skills within nursing, it is clear that it is nursing that is called to account in the first place. The debate about the expanded role of the nurse is then sharpened and focused, and rightly so, but so are other aspects, in particular the role of the relationship between nurses and clients, and whether this is a partnership or a contractual arrangement. In either case, good supervision for counselling practice is not only advisable, but essential.

Nurses as agents of change

Whenever you influence something, you change it. Egan (1994, p. 58) suggests that 'helping is a social-influence process even though it is still not clear how it works.' He quotes Driscoll (1984) who said that 'the obvious objective of helping is not merely to understand, but to benefit troubled persons. The emphasis is thus on influence, and on the concepts, understanding, procedures and competencies used to generate changes'.

All of helping is a challenge to clients (see Chapter 9) and there has to be some change at the end of a helping interaction, otherwise there has been no 'helping'. As helping does not mean imposing or demanding something, but fostering the client's self-helping abilities and skills, helpers are inevitably agents of change. But they are this also as nurses, doctors and carers of many disciplines. The ways suggested in this book to promote and use the skills of helping should be one means of being effective change agents.

Some of the ways in which human skills are taught and learnt in nursing is to consider 'partnership in caring'. This involves demonstrating effective communication skill, acting as advocate for the patient or client, managing conflict constructively, and showing assertiveness in action. These are essentially the skills of effective agents of change: people who do not accept the status quo simply because someone said so, or because they are too timid; people who so passionately care for others that they will speak up for them; people who strive for a better environment wherever this is possible by uncovering conflict and facing it constructively.

These are not easy issues to tackle. The essence of all interaction between nurses and patients must ultimately rest on the relationship and on human rights, *not* human wants, but real, fundamental human needs (Curtin, 1979).

Nurses as advocates

Curtin (1979) bases the concept of advocacy in

the basic nature and purpose of the nurse–patient relationship, which in turn is based upon our common humanity, our common needs and our common human rights. We are human beings, our patients or clients are human beings, and it is this commonality that should form the basis of the relationship between us.

A dictionary definition of an advocate may be one who pleads for another. The nurse as advocate pleads the cause of the patient. Unfortunately, this has largely come to mean fighting the 'system'. In the above terms advocacy is more subtle and concerns *human values*.

According to Brown (1985), there are four broad areas where patient advocacy is called for; these correspond largely to the principles of ethics outlined above: (1) in the quality of care which patients receive (the principles of the value of life, and of goodness and right); (2) in the right and access to care which patients should have (the principle of justice and fairness); (3) in full information which they should receive (the principle of truth telling and honesty); and (4) in the area of alternatives to care (the principle of individual freedom). Brown suspects that 'too often, the only alternative offered to treatment is no treatment. The patient is thus faced with making an impossible decision'.

When patients have received full information, they may not need someone who pleads their cause, but someone who gives them the opportunity to discover, explore and clarify the alternatives, not only to treatments but to living and coping generally, so that through them they can live more resourcefully and satisfyingly.

The reverse may be more often the case: a nurse discovers, through counselling, that a patient is not receiving quality of care, or the full information, or is not involved enough in the process of care, and the nurse then becomes the patient's advocate. In that sense advocacy may become 'fighting the system'.

Walsh (1985) points out that nurses who act as advocates have the problem of a split in loyalties:

When a nurse takes on the role of advocate she must consider not only the patient, but her own career, her relationship with the doctor, and the need of her employer. Being an advocate is not a neutral role.

Walsh goes on to say that many nurses would see it as the ultimate objective to lead patients to 'self-advocacy', possibly through pressure groups. Self-advocacy thus coincides with the concept of self-responsibility and having the necessary self-help skills, where clients set their own goals and strive to achieve them.

Confidentiality

Bond (1993, p. 204) makes a strong point for confidentiality:

A counsellor's practice of confidentiality is closely associated with considerations of client autonomy. Confidentiality acts like a fence round the space created for the client's autonomous actions. The fence is important to the client's safety and creates the circumstances in which clients can look at issues which otherwise would be kept to themselves. The fence also marks a boundary of responsibility. Care over confidentiality reinforces the client's sense of responsibility for the outcome of the counselling. Therefore confidentiality is extremely important in counselling. Care over confidentiality is a practical way of signalling respect for a client's autonomy.

Unless patients and clients know that they can trust their helpers, they are unlikely to talk about themselves. Sometimes you may need to give patients the assurance beforehand that anything said between you is indeed between you only. If possible, you should then ensure that no one else overhears, something not so easily achieved in, for example, a hospital ward.

There are numerous occasions when clients are rightly concerned that any information they give to nurses and helpers might leak to families and friends with disastrous consequences. For whatever reason, some clients cannot or dare not (or at least not yet) be open about their diagnoses or about certain tests they are having. Or the fact that someone has been receiving counselling may be wrongly interpreted by someone with a vested interest. Hospital wards, dining rooms and buses seem at times to have ears all round, and have all been the scene of unwitting disclosures by nurses not aware of their duty to keep matters confidential.

Most of the time what is said between helper and client is not particularly confidential, but it is not idle talk. Simply the fact that what has been discussed does not go further is reassuring. Occasionally you may hear disturbing facts related by patients. There may be some very good reasons why individuals chose to reveal a certain aspect of themselves, or a deed they have done. Not only do you have to be unshockable, but sometimes you also have to live with disturbing knowledge. This is yet another reason for good and regular supervision.

Occasionally it is not possible, for one reason or another, to keep something confidential. It is then not only courteous but essential that the client knows what you are going to do, and that such an action is consented to.

Record keeping

It is becoming more and more usual for patients to see their case notes or to take part in hand-over reports. What is said and written has, therefore, not only to be accurate, but actually helpful to the patient.

To say (or write) that you had a talk with a patient is often helpful because it may make your relationship legitimate in the eyes of your colleagues. It may also help the other members of staff to respect your relationship with that particular patient. And knowing that you are the patient's 'counsellor' may indeed relieve other colleagues from a sense of duty, by knowing that one of their number has taken that aspect seriously. How much you record of the content of such a conversation is up to you and the client concerned.

Anyone who helps clients on a regular basis will need to keep some form of record. This is not only for your memory, but shows also a respect for clients and the work they have put into a session. Keeping records is time-consuming and there has to be some system in place for it. As with hospital records, patients and clients should have access to the records kept about them. However, others, such as employers or supervisors, would need to make a very strong case before they should be given access to personal records. Some supervisors may want counsellors to work with them from their records.

Bond (1993, p. 177) gives some examples of the type of records that counsellors might use, but he also says that it is difficult to know what is good practice (p. 165) in record keeping.

Conflicting interests

There are numerous occasions when interests conflict. The principle of truth telling may conflict with the idea of respect for the person: should the truth win, or the comfort of the patient? The institution that employs you does so in good faith and you consider that helping and counselling a few people is more important than bathing every patient. But a manager questions who gave you the permission just to talk. Your values and your professional judgement are questioned. Which wins, or who wins? Is it the one against the many?

There are no guidelines that can be laid down for such circumstances. Part of the challenge of ethics is that such problems and dilemmas can and are dealt with in a fitting way which is right and good and enhancing the humanity of all concerned.

Counselling and the institution

Most nurses who have and use counselling skills work in institutions or agencies of one kind or another. And, since counselling is a social-influence process, by sheer dint of *doing* counselling they influence people and systems around them. Yet many nurses find that their organization is 'alienating', i.e. it is a 'social order which is "remote", incomprehensible or fraudulent; beyond hope or desire; inviting apathy, boredom or even hostility' (Nisbet, 1969). It is hardly surprising that many nurses see their organization as something that is against them; therefore they can only be against it in return. Yet, because they work in it, they also need it and use it.

Jameton (1984, p. 6) talks of moral problems in nursing, and reserves the strongest type, moral distress, for situations 'when one knows the right thing to do, but institutional constraints make it nearly impossible to pursue the right course of action'.

When using counselling skills openly with patients and colleagues you may come in conflict with the organization. Or the institution, through its senior personnel, may feel that you are doing something that is not strictly in your job description, and for which permission has not been given. Either way, there is conflict, and eventually distress.

But counselling and helping are also seen as more and more important elements in nursing. Alone you cannot change the institution to subscribe to this form of care; but you can influence the institution.

When you believe that using counselling and helping skills in health care settings is better than not using them, not only will individual patients benefit, but the system itself will become less alienating, less remote, more comprehensible, more caring and more contented. As you cannot do this single-handedly, you need to do it in a way which the organization understands.

Just as your clients will have gained self-helping skills by the end of the counselling you have done, so you also have the same capabilities and opportunities. As a nurse you can influence the system by promoting counselling, seeking the skills, acquiring them and using them. Thus, counselling has come full circle.

Ethical issues are not something extra or different from helping and caring in general. The caring nurse is inevitably an ethical nurse, and vice versa. What may be new is the language of some of the concepts. What remains is that at the centre there is a person with needs – and that could be you one day, which may be a sobering thought in terms of duty, or responsibility, and your response to suffering in general.

CHAPTER FIFTEEN

Resources

....

Learning on your own

Since counselling is an interpersonal process, it is also learnt interpersonally. Books and articles are therefore of only limited use. Nevertheless, there are many excellent books available covering many different areas and aspects of counselling.

A literature search in any library will quickly reveal many titles, and give an idea of possible areas for further study.

Writing to publishers for their catalogues can also be helpful, since they annotate most titles and thus give useful information of the content of particular books.

A librarian would also be helpful with information contained in books.

In the UK, the Library of the Royal College of Nursing has a good stock of books on counselling. They also have a literature search and photocopying service.

> The Library (Information)
> Royal College of Nursing
> 20 Cavendish Square
> London W1M 0AB
> Telephone: 0171 499 3333

Meditec, the Medical and Nursing Booksellers, have a comprehensive catalogue of the books they stock and sell. They are specialists in mail-order services and there is no charge for posting.

> Meditec Medical and Nursing Booksellers
> Jackson's Yard
> Brewery Hill
> Grantham
> Lincs, NG31 6DW
> Telephone: 01476 590 505
> Fax: 01476 590 329

Among the books referred to in this volume, the following are particularly recommended for further reading:

Barker, P.J. (1993) *A Self-Help Guide to Managing Depression*. London: Chapman and Hall.

This is a slim volume specifically written for people who are depressed. Helpers will find this book useful, either for recommending it to depressed people or for using its guidelines in their work with people suffering from depression.

Berne, E. (1964) *Games People Play*. Harmondsworth: Penguin.

This is an old favourite for understanding the many different plays or 'scripts' that people use in everyday life and interactions.

Burnard, P. (1994) *Counselling Skills for Health Professionals* (2nd edn). London: Chapman and Hall.

This second edition of Burnard's text is greatly expanded and includes a useful section on the theory of psychology at the beginning.

Dryden, W. (1994) *Overcoming Guilt*. London: Sheldon.

Dryden has written very accessibly on the subject of guilt, which comes up again and again in counselling. Guilt is a notoriously difficult subject to get to grips with, and this little book goes a long way to make it more understandable.

Egan, G. (1994) *The Skilled Helper* (5th edn). Belmont, California: Brooks/Cole Publishing.

Egan's regular updates of his book are most helpful. His style is clear and he uses examples for every detail that he describes. It is a book for counsellors, and people using counselling skills (rather than being counsellors) may find it too detailed. Nevertheless, this book should be on the shelf (and used) by all who do any counselling.

MacLean, D. & Gould, S. (1988) *The Helping Process: An Introduction*. Beckenham: Croom Helm.

These authors describe the process of helping very well; the bulk of the book concentrates on the beginning, middle and ending of the helping relationship.

Mearns, D. & Thorne, B. (1988) *Person-centred Counselling in Action*. London: Sage.

This is one of the 'Counselling in Action' series by Sage, which is excellent. The theories of Rogers are described and detailed.

Murgatroyd, S. (1985) *Counselling and Helping*. Leicester: British Psychological Society; and London: Routledge.

This is a good text for people using counselling skills, as it concentrates on the 'helping' aspects of the activities.

Nelson-Jones, R. (1982) *The Theory and Practice of Counselling Psychology*. London: Cassell.

The title of this comprehensive and meticulously compiled book of over 530 pages speaks for itself: there is basic theory and psychology, and for anyone interested in studying counselling in depth this is a most useful text.

Nelson-Jones, R. (1993) *Practical Counselling and Helping Skills* (3rd edn). London: Cassell.

Nelson-Jones concentrates on the life-skills model of helping in this book, which is packed full of information often not included by other authors. Unfortunately, the print is not easy to read, especially in the practical examples.

Rogers, C.R. (1961) *On Becoming a Person*. London: Constable.

This is perhaps Rogers' best known book. It is written from a personal perspective and is a 'must' for every serious counsellor. Rogers was more of a philosopher in his writings and this is particularly evident in this early volume.

Rogers, C.R. (1980) *A Way of Being*. Boston: Houghton Mifflin.

This was Rogers' last work and describes empathy in the way only Rogers could bring it alive.

Scrutton, S. (1989) *Counselling Older People*. London: Edward Arnold.

As many nurses and helpers will come in contact with elderly people who call on them for help, this practical book is worth a read.

Stewart, W. (1992) *An A–Z of Counselling Theory and Practice*. London: Chapman and Hall.

This is a compilation of all the main theories and practices in lists and headings, and will be particularly helpful for those who need to write essays (and books!) on counselling.

Tschudin, V. (1994) *Counselling. A Primer for Nurses. Workbook and Workshop Guide*. London: Baillière Tindall.

The various packages in this series are designed for use in workshops, but the Workbooks are meant to be read by participants beforehand, and worked through on their own. They are therefore very practical and ideal for learning on one's own.

Worden, J.W. (1994) *Grief Counselling and Grief Therapy* (2nd edn). London: Scutari.

This is a classic text, specifically written for mental health practitioners, but ideal for any health care professional. The second, updated, edition is not only a resource, but valuable in the whole area of bereavement counselling and help.

Courses

There is almost a bewildering array of courses available to anyone wanting to learn counselling. It is therefore difficult to know which is the course best suited to your own requirements. The titles of courses do not necessarily correspond to what is taught. It is therefore always wise to check what the content and philosophy of a course is before embarking on it. It is also helpful to know whether you are looking for a course that teaches counselling skills, or that trains participants to be counsellors. People who have done a few weekend courses are not either able or qualified to call themselves 'counsellors'. The minimum requirement for a qualification to practice under the title 'counsellor' is 450 hours (British Association for Counselling, 1994c).

The British Association for Counselling leaflet 'Training in Counselling' has useful information and also lists courses.

The notice-boards of libraries, town halls and universities are useful places for advertising and finding courses in counselling. Personal contact with people who have either completed a course or who are trained counsellors is perhaps the best starting point for finding out about courses.

For information about courses contact:

British Association for Counselling
1 Regent Place
Rugby CV21 2PJ

Telephone: 01788 550 899 (office)
01788 578 328 (information line)
Fax: 0178 562 189

Accreditation

The British Association for Counselling operates an accreditation scheme for individual counsellors and a recognition scheme for counselling courses and supervisors. It is the only national organization to do this.

Accreditation is not necessary for the practice of counselling, but more and more qualified counsellors seek accreditation, and institutions employing counsellors normally demand accreditation. When looking for courses, or when thinking of counselling as a career, it is useful to consider working towards accreditation.

Accreditation with the British Association for Counselling demands regular supervised practice, and practitioners have to renew accreditation regularly. It is therefore not a one-off event and this assures the highest standards possible. Some counsellors find this too demanding, particularly when they have small case-loads.

Postscript

To arrive at the end of a book is always an anti-climax – pleased to be there, and wondering, is it alright?

So I am left with the question, is it clear, will the readers understand it? Will it help them? I have written that counselling is for better or for worse; the same can apply to a book. Will it contribute to make practice better or worse? Being an optimist, of course I hope that it will make practice better.

I should be able to apply the self-helping skills outlined to myself. I should know how to monitor myself and have enough awareness to judge the book and know that, if there are mistakes, that is not all there is to it. Sometimes the position of author and 'expert' frightens me. Are not you, the reader, the expert? I learn a great deal from simple conversations with friends and the people I counsel. A friend who is having a great number of family problems just now, told me yesterday, 'I have done so much psychodrama over the years; now I am actually living it'. I can echo this: I have written so much over the years, I too, have to live it. Perhaps that is the message I would now like to hand on: we have to live it.

However much we are expert at certain things, there will always be points of doubt and uncertainty. These are the moments when we need help. It need not be a complete analysis before we can function again, but the basic needs of being acknowledged as human beings and assured of our worth as the person we are. This is done only when we are listened to.

Readers who know of my twin interests of counselling and ethics know also that I have often said and written that if I could add one right to the many rights that people are more and more claiming, it would be the right to be listened to. At the end of this book I would like to say it again: we should have a right to be listened to, and this means in return a responsibility to listen to others. It means also a need to listen to ourselves and to our needs. The self-awareness with which this book began is therefore also the end of it.

Bibliography

Altschul, A. & Sinclair, H.C. (1981) *Psychology for Nurses*. London: Baillière Tindall.

Bailey, B., Claveirole, A., MacKenzie, C. & Wright, M. (1994) An educational support group. *Nursing Standard* **8**(30): 65–57, 71, 73.

Bailey, R. (1981) Counselling services for nurses – a forgotten responsibility. *Apex (Journal of the British Institute of Mental Handicap)* **9**(2): 45–47.

Bandler, R. (1985) *Using your Brain – For a Change*. Moab, Utah: Real People Press.

Barker, P.J. (1993) *A Self-Help Guide to Managing Depression*. London: Chapman and Hall.

Bayne, R., Horton, I., Merry, T. & Noyes, E. (1994) *The Counsellor's Handbook*. London: Chapman and Hall.

Beauchamp, T.L. & Childress, J.F. (1989) *Principles of Biomedical Ethics* (3rd edn). New York: Oxford University Press.

Benjamin, M. & Curtis, J. (1986) *Ethics in Nursing* (2nd edn). New York: Oxford University Press.

Berne, E. (1964) *Games People Play*. Harmondsworth: Penguin.

Bond, T. (1993) *Standards and Ethics for Counselling in Action*. London: Sage.

Booth, P. (1985) Back on the rails. *Nursing Times* **81**(35): 16–17.

British Association for Counselling (1989) *Code of Ethics and Practice for Counselling Skills*. Rugby: BAC.

British Association for Counselling (1993) *Code of Ethics and Practice for Counsellors*. Rugby: BAC.

British Association for Counselling (1994a) *Counselling – Some Questions Answered* (leaflet). Rugby: BAC.

British Association for Counselling (1994b). News item. *Counselling* **5**(4): 252–253.

British Association for Counselling (1994c) *Training in counselling* (leaflet TrPk4/94). Rugby: BAC

Brown, M. (1985) Matter of commitment. *Nursing Times* **81**(18): 26–27.

Brown, J. (1988) Care of the dying. In Tschudin, V. (ed.) *Nursing the Patient with Cancer*. Hemel Hempstead: Prentice Hall, pp. 409–424.

Buckroyd, J. & Smith, E. (1990) Learning to help. *Nursing Times* **86**(35): 54–57.

Burnard, P. (1990a) Stating the case. *Counselling* November: 114–116.

Burnard, P. (1990b) Counselling the boss. *Nursing Times* **86**(1): 58–59.

Burnard, P. (1994) *Counselling Skills for Health Professionals* (2nd edn). London: Chapman and Hall.

Burton, G. (1979) *Interpersonal Relations, a Guide for Nurses*. London: Tavistock.

Butterworth, C.A. & Faugier, J. (1994) *Clinical Supervision. A position paper*. Manchester: University of Manchester.

Carkhuff, R.R. (1987) *The Art of Helping* (6th edn). Amherst: Human Resource Development Press.

Castledine, G. (1994) What is clinical supervision? *British Journal of Nursing* **3**(21): 1135.

Chambers Dictionary (1993) Edinburgh: Chambers Harrap.

Charnock, A. (1985) Sharing the sadness. *Nursing Times* **81**(40): 40–41.

Clarke, L. (1986) Deterioration effects induced by psychological counselling. *Counselling* **57**: 8–13.

Cormack, D. (1985) The myth and reality of interpersonal skills use in nursing. In Kagan, C.M. (ed.) (1985) *Interpersonal Skills in Nursing*. London: Croom Helm.

Crawley, P. (1983) Call in for a chat. *Nursing Mirror* **156**(14): 510.

Curtin, L.L. (1979) The nurse as advocate: a philosophical foundation for nursing. *Advances in Nursing Science* **1**(3): 1–10.

Daniel, J. (1984) 'Sympathy' or 'empathy'? *Journal of Medical Ethics* **10**(2): 103 (letter).

Davies, M. (1993) Counselling; a statistical analysis within the primary health care team. *Counselling in Medical Settings News* (37): 5–10.

Davis, K. (1972) In Lancaster, J. & Lancaster, W. (1982) *Concepts for Advanced Nursing Practice*. St Louis: C.V. Mosby.

Doust, M. (1991) Student nurses and counselling services. *Nursing Standard* **5**(1): 35–37.

Dowrick, S. (1993) *The Intimacy and Solitude Self-Therapy Book*. London: The Women's Press.

Driscoll, R. (1984) Pragmatic psychotherapy. New York: Van Nostrand Reinhold.

Dryden, W. (1994) *Overcoming Guilt*. London: Sheldon.

Duncan, A.S., Dunstan, G.R. & Wellbourn, R.B. (1981) *Dictionary of Medical Ethics* (2nd edn). London: Darton, Longman & Todd.

Egan, G. (1977) *You and Me*. Monterey, CA: Brooks/Cole.

Egan, G. (1986) *The Skilled Helper* (3rd edn). Belmont, CA: Wadsworth.

Egan, G. (1994) *The Skilled Helper* (5th edn). Belmont, CA: Brooks/Cole.

Ellis, A. (1962) *Reason and Emotion in Psychotherapy*. New York: Lyle Stuart.

Eliot, T.S. (1944) *Four Quartets*. London: Faber & Faber.

Erikson, E.H. (1964) *Childhood and Society* (revised edn). Harmondsworth: Penguin.

Fabun, D. (1968) Communications. Beverley Hills: Glencoe Press.

Faugier, J. (1991) Elected to counsel. *Nursing Times* **87**(46): 22.

Ferrucci, P. (1982) *What We May Be*. Wellingborough: Thorsons.

Forsyth, G.L. (1979) Exploration of empathy in nurse–client interaction. *Advances in Nursing Science* **1**(2): 53–61.

Fox, J. (1994) Clinical supervision: a real aspiration? *British Journal of Nursing* **3**(16): 805.

Frankl, V. (1962) *Man's Search for Meaning*. London: Hodder & Stoughton.

Fraser, J. (1990) Reading between the lines. *Nursing Times* **86**(5): 45–47.

Fromant, P. (1988) Helping each other. *Nursing Times* **84**(36): 30, 32.

Gawain, S. (1978) *Creative Visualization*. New York: Bantam.

Gilbert, P. (1989) *Human Nature and Suffering*. Hove: Lawrence Erlbaum.

Glasser, W. (1965) *Reality Therapy*. New York: Harper & Row.

Goldman, E.E. & Morrison, D.S. (1984) *Psychodrama: Experience and Process*. Dubuque, IA: Kendall/Hunt.

Harris, T.A. (1973) *I'm OK – You're OK*. London: Pan Books.

Heywood Jones, I. (1989) Buried under paper. *Nursing Times* **85**(34): 57–58.

Hore, I.D. (1984) Can managers counsel? *Counselling* **48**: 7–13.

Hough, M. (1994) *A Practical Approach to Counselling*. London: Pitman.

Jacobs, M. (1982) *Still Small Voice*. London: Society for Promoting Christian Knowledge.

Jameton, A. (1984) *Nursing Practice: the Ethical Issues*. Englewood Cliffs, NJ: Prentice-Hall.

Jung, C.G. (1964) *Man and his Symbols*. London: Pan.

Kalisch, B.J. (1971) Strategies for developing nurse empathy. *Nursing Outlook* **19**(11): 714–717.

King, J. (1984) A question of attitude. *Nursing Times* **80**(45): 51–52.

Kirkpatrick, W. (1985) *Reaching Out*. Private circulation.

Kohner, N. (1994) *Clinical Supervision in Practice*. London: King's Fund Centre.

Krumboltz, J.D. & Thorenson, C.E. (1969) *Behavioral counselling: cases and techniques*. New York: Holt, Rinehart & Winston.

Kübler-Ross, E. (1969) *On Death and Dying*. London: Tavistock.

Lomas, P. (1994) *Cultivating Intuition*. London: Penguin.

MacLean, D. & Gould, S. (1988) *The Helping Process: An Introduction*. Beckenham: Croom Helm.

Macleod Clark, J., Hopper, L. & Jesson, A. (1991) Progression to Counselling. *Nursing Times* **87**(8): 41–43.

Marks, R. & Hingley, P. (1991) *The Cost of Stress and the Benefits of Stress Management*. Occasional Paper No. 5. Woking: National Association for Staff Support.

Marks-Maran, D. (1993) Accountability. In Tschudin, V. (ed.) *Ethics: Nurses and Patients*. London: Scutari, pp. 121–134.

Martin, I.C.A. (1977) A strident silence. *Nursing Times* **73**(19): 754–755.

Mathews, B.P. (1962) Measurement of psychological aspects of the nurse–patient relationship. *Nursing Research* **11**(3): 154–162.

Mayeroff, M. (1971) *On Caring*. New York: Harper & Row.

Mearns, D. & Thorne, B. (1988) *Person-centred Counselling in Action*. London: Sage.

Meize-Grochowski, R. (1984) An analysis of the concept of trust. *Journal of Advanced Nursing* **9**: 563–572.

Menzies, I. (1960) A case-study in the functioning of social systems as a defence against anxiety. *Human Relations* **13**(2): 95–121.

Miller, W.A. (1981) *Make Friends with Your Shadow*. Minneapolis, MN: Augsburg Publishing.

Murgatroyd, S. (1985) *Counselling and Helping*. Leicester: British Psychological Society; and London: Routledge.

National Association for Staff Support (1992) *A Charter for Staff Support*. Woking: National Association for Staff Support.

National Association for Staff Support (1994) *Newslink* September: 1.

Navone, J. (1977) *Towards a Theology of Story*. Slough: St Paul Publications.

Nelson-Jones, R. (1982) *The Theory and Practice of Counselling Psychology*. London: Cassell.

Nelson-Jones, R. (1993) *Practical Counselling and Helping Skills* (3rd edn). London: Cassell.

Nisbet, R. (1969) *The Quest for Community*. London: Oxford University Press, p. 9.

Nouwen, H.J., McNeill, D.P. & Morrison, D.A. (1982) *Compassion*. London: Darton, Longman & Todd.

Nurse, G. (1978) What is counselling? *Midwife, Health Visitor and Community Nurse* **14**(10): 352–355.

Nurse, G. (1980) *Counselling and the Nurse* (2nd edn). Aylesbury: HM & M.

Nursing Standard (1994) News: NHS managers urged to help staff cope with stress at work. *Nursing Standard* **8**(19): 9.

Ogier, M. & Cameron-Buccheri, R. (1990) Supervision: a cross-cultural approach. *Nursing Standard* **4**(31): 24–26.

Owen, G. (1993) *Taking the Strain*. Literature Review (5th edn). Woking: National Association for Staff Support.

Peck, M.S. (1993) *A World Waiting to be Born*. London: Arrow Books.

Perls, F. (1973) *The Gestalt Approach and Eye Witness to Therapy*. New York: Bantam.

Perry, F. (1988) Far from black and white. *Nursing Times* **84**(10): 40–41.

Philips, J. (1993) Counselling and the nurse. *British Journal of Theatre Nursing* **2**(10): 13–14.

Quilliam, S. (1991) When empathy gets dangerous. *Practice Nurse* **4**(5): 305–306, 312.

Riley, V.A. (1983) Counselling the mentally handicapped. *Counselling* **43**: 10–13.

Roach, M.S. (1985) Caring as responsivity: a response to value as the important-in-itself. Paper delivered at the 2nd International Congress on Nursing Law and Ethics, Tel Aviv, June 1985.

Roach, M.S. (1992) *The Human Act of Caring: A Blueprint for the Health Professions* (rev. edn). Ottawa: Canadian Hospital Association.

Rogers, C.R. (1951) *Client-Centred Therapy*. Boston: Houghton Mifflin.

Rogers, C.R. (1957) Empathic: an unappreciated way of being. *Counselling Psychologist* **12**: 95–103.

Rogers, C.R. (1961) *On Becoming a Person*. London: Constable.

Rogers, C.R. (1967) *The Therapeutic Relationship and its Impact*. Madison: University of Wisconsin.

Rogers, C.R. (1978) *On Personal Power*. London: Constable.

Rogers, C.R. (1980) *A Way of Being.* Boston: Houghton Mifflin.

Salvage, J. (1990) The theory and practice of the 'new nursing'. *Nursing Times,* occasional paper **86**(1): 42–45.

Schön, D.A. (1987) *Educating the Reflective Practitioner.* London: Jossey-Bass.

Scrutton, S. (1989) *Counselling Older People.* London: Edward Arnold.

Simonton, S., Simonton, O.C. & Creighton, J.C. (1978) *Getting Well Again.* New York: Bantam.

Smith, K. (1994) A lifetime of opportunity. *Nursing Times* **90**(44): 14–15.

Smith, P. (1989) Nurses' emotional labour. *Nursing Times* **85**(47): 49–51.

Speck, P. (1992) Managing the boundaries. *Nursing Times* **88**(32): 22.

Stewart, W. (1992) *An A–Z of Counselling Theory and Practice.* London: Chapman and Hall.

Taylor, J.V. (1972) *The Go-Between God.* London: SCM Press.

Thiroux, J. (1980) *Ethics: Theory and Practice* (2nd edn). Encino, CA: Glencoe Publishing.

Tomlinson, A. (1983) *Communication Skills: Questioning.* Private circulation.

Truax, C.B. (1961) A scale for the measurement of accurate empathy. *Psychiatric Institute Bulletin*, University of Wisconsin **1**: 12.

Truax, C.B. & Carkhuff, R.R. (1967) *Towards Effective Counselling and Psychotherapy.* Chicago: Aldine.

Tschudin, V. (1981) A question of mind over matter? *Nursing Times* **77**(10): 424–426.

Tschudin, V. (1989a) Ethics, morality and nursing. In Hinchliff, S.M., Norman, S.E. & Schober, J.E. (eds) (1989) *Nursing Practice and Health Care.* London: Edward Arnold, pp. 328–343.

Tschudin, V. (1989b) *Beginning with Empathy. A facilitator's guide.* Edinburgh: Churchill Livingstone.

Tschudin, V. (1989c) *Beginning with Empathy. A learner's handbook.* Edinburgh: Churchill Livingstone.

Tschudin, V. (1991) *Beginning with Awareness. A learner's handbook and facilitator's guide.* Edinburgh: Churchill Livingstone.

Tschudin, V. (1992) *Values. A Primer for Nurses. Workbook and Workshop Guide.* London: Baillière Tindall.

Tschudin, V. (1994) *Counselling. A Primer for Nurses. Workbook and Workshop Guide.* London: Baillière Tindall.

Tschudin, V. & Marks-Maran, D. (1993) *Ethics. A Primer for*

Nurses. Workbook and Workshop Guide. London: Baillière Tindall.

United Kingdom Central Council (1992) *Code of Professional Conduct for the Nurse, Midwife and Health Visitor* (3rd edn). London: UKCC.

Walsh, P. (1985) Speaking up for the patient. *Nursing Times* **81**(18): 24–27.

Wells, R. (1988) Ethics and Informed Consent. In Tschudin, V. (ed.) *Nursing the Patient with Cancer*. Hemel Hempstead: Prentice Hall, pp. 459–475.

Worden, J.W. (1983) *Grief Counselling and Grief Therapy; A Handbook for the Mental Health Practitioner*. London: Routledge.

Index